FLOWER ESSENCES

AN ILLUSTRATED GUIDE

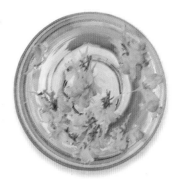

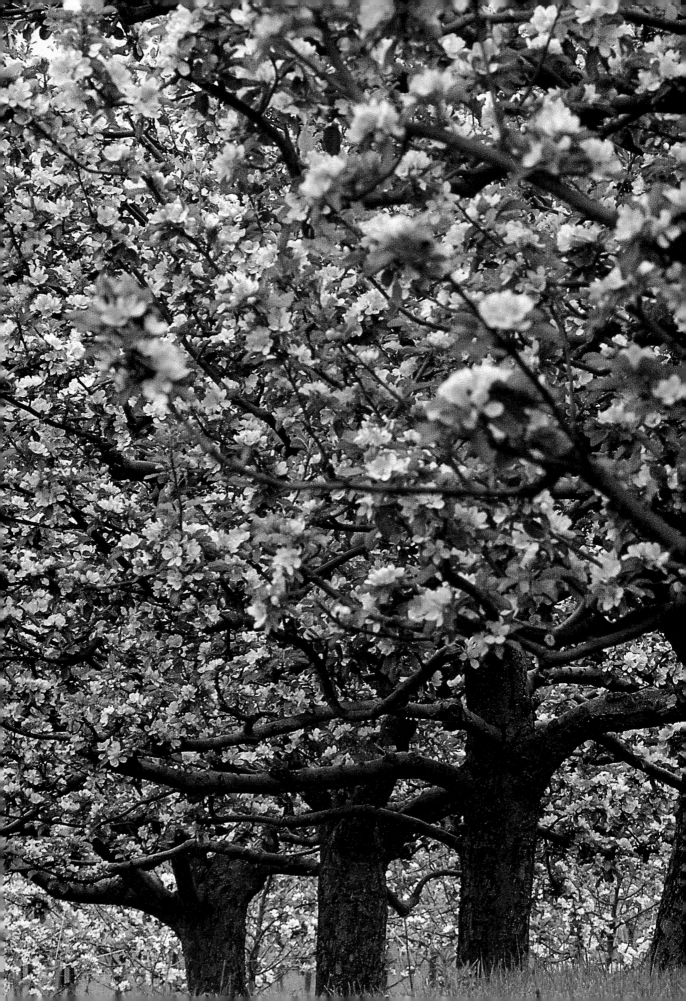

FLOWER ESSENCES
AN ILLUSTRATED GUIDE

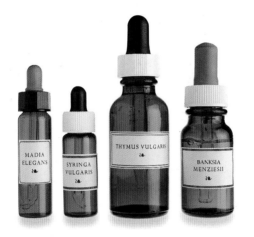

CAROL RUDD

Shaftesbury, Dorset • Boston, Massachusetts • Melbourne, Victoria

© Element Books Limited 1998

First published in Great Britain in 1998 by
ELEMENT BOOKS LIMITED
Shaftesbury, Dorset, SP7 9BP

Published in the USA in 1998 by
ELEMENT BOOKS INC
160 North Washington Street, Boston, MA 02114

Published in Australia in 1998 by
ELEMENT BOOKS
and distributed by Penguin Australia Ltd
487 Maroondah Highway, Ringwood, Victoria 3134

Reprinted 1999

NOTE FROM THE PUBLISHER
*Any information given in this book is not intended to be taken
as a replacement for medical advice. Any person with a condition
requiring medical attention should consult a qualified
practitioner or therapist.*

Designed and created with
THE BRIDGEWATER BOOK COMPANY LIMITED

ELEMENT BOOKS LIMITED
Editorial Director: JULIA MCCUTCHEN
Senior Commissioning Editor: CARO NESS
Production Director: ROGER LANE
Production: SARAH GOLDEN

THE BRIDGEWATER BOOK COMPANY
Art Director: KEVIN KNIGHT
Designer: JANE LANAWAY
Page makeup: CHRIS LANAWAY
Managing Editor: ANNE TOWNLEY
Project Editor: CAROLINE EARLE
Project Manager: JULIE WHITAKER
Picture Research: LYNDA MARSHALL
Three-dimensional models: MARK JAMIESON
Studio photography: ANNE HYDE, WALTER GARDINER PHOTOGRAPHY
Additional photography: IAN PARSONS, GUY RYECART
Illustrations: LORRAINE HARRISON, JOANNE MAKIN, MOIRA WILLS
Scientific illustrations: MICHAEL COURTENEY

Repro by Appletone Graphics, Bournemouth, England.

Printed by
Graphicom Srl, Vicenza, Italy.

British Library Cataloguing in Publication
data available

Library of Congress Cataloging-in-Publication data available

Acknowledgments

*The publisher would like to thank
the following for the use of pictures:*
Alaskan Flower Essence Project, Homer: 52b (Steve Johnson).
Aloha, Hawaiian Tropical Flower Essences, Kealakekua: 34b.
Ancient Art & Architecture Collection, London: 27b, 65t, 73b.
Australian Bush Essences, Dee Why, NSW: 40b, 54b, 58b, 104l.
Australian Flower Essence Academy, Perth: 30b, 46b, 48l, 80l.
A–Z Botanical Collection, London: 44b, 94.
Bridgeman Art Library, London: 9t (Christie's, London);
30t (City of Bristol Museum & Art Galleries); 63b (Library of Congress,
Washington); 69b (National Gallery, London); 71t (V&A, London);
91b (Fratelli Fabbri, Milan); 93t (Private Collection); 99b (Fitzwilliam
Museum, University of Cambridge); 100b, 103 (National Gallery, Scotland);
111 (Valley of the Kings, Thebes); 115 (Palazzo Vecchio, Florence).
Corbis Bettmann/UPI, London: 53t, 95l.
Desert Alchemy, Tucson: 38l (Camilio Scherer).
e.t. archive, London: 13, 23t, 25r, 33t, 59, 63t, 84t, 87, 105l, 107l, 113b.
Flower Essence Society, Nevada: 24br, 82.
Garden Picture Library, London: 2 (Robert Estall); 34t (Lamontagne);
37t, 70l (J. S. Sira); 56b (Howard Rice); 72 (Christopher Gallagher);
98l (Brigitte Thomas); 101 (Phil Jude).
Harry Smith Collection, Essex: 36r.
Healing Herbs, Hereford: 86l (Julian Barnard).
Image Bank, London: 14b, 49, 50t.
Pacific Essences®, Victoria, British Columbia: 28l (S. Pettitt).
Robert Harding Picture Library, London: 117t.
Rudolf Steiner House, London: 9b.
Science Photo Library, London: 12tl, 12r.
Zefa UK/Stock Market, London: 16r, 28t, 31t, 39t, 47t, 55, 64br, 75t,
77c, 78t, 81b, 89t, 95t, 109t.

Special thanks to:
Patricia Blunt, Robert Chappell, Rukshana Chenoy, Jessie Fuller,
Cathy Glendinning, Andrew Harley, Eleanor Harley, Mary Harley,
Jill Howell and her dog, Kevin Irvine, Mette Wiese Lauritzen, Denise
McCullough, Caron Riley, Vincent Riley, Laurel Scrace, Sheila Sword,
Amelia Whitelaw, Gabriel Whitelaw
for help with the photography

Authors' Acknowledgments

*I would like to thank my husband, Chris Rudd;
the Essence & Energy Flower Group (Tess, Val, Lynne, Flic);
the Pentad (Tess, Jutta, Bee & Liz); Gayle;
Richard Katz & Patricia Kaminski; my clients for material for the case studies;
Judy Griffin for part of the Zinnia case study;
Simon Lilly for the Lilac and Ash case histories;
Liz; and my editor, Caro Ness.*

ISBN 1 86204 167 9

Contents

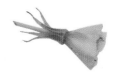

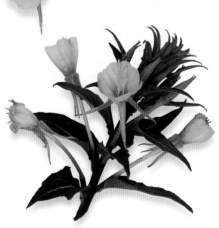

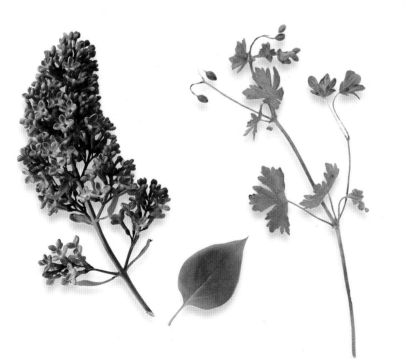

Introduction

A FLOWER ESSENCE *is the essential healing energy of a flower, the distinctive dynamic inner life force that differentiates it from other flowers. As we capture the juices and oils from the leaves, stems, and roots of plants to make herbal medicines for the body, so we can utilize the more subtle energy of the bloom for mental, emotional, and spiritual healing. A plant's bloom contains the generative energy needed for its reproduction. Moreover, when a plant is in flower this energy is expressed in its color and an infinite variety of wonderful shapes. It is at the peak of its beauty.*

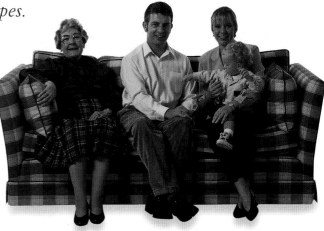

ABOVE *Flower essences can be used to treat old and young, male and female.*

Each flower has its own special effect, depending on the "character" of the plant. A flower essence may calm you, energize you, make you more tolerant, or help you to be more assertive. Flower essence therapy is natural healing. Many of us are cut off from nature. However, when we decide to take a flower essence rather than a painkiller, we give ourselves a natural "dose" of the beauty of the plant world. This influences the quality of our thoughts, which can then filter down into the body to heal us. There are many flower essence formulas available now that need only a little knowledge for them to be used with great effect. Animals as well as humans can benefit from flower essences. Administer the essences in the same dosages as you would for humans. Plants also thrive on essences. A plant that has been transplanted will adapt more easily to its new environment if given some drops of walnut to support it. Giving a plant a remedy in its water will enhance its life force, whatever that essence may be.

LEFT *Add Chicory flower essence to a whining dog's drinking water to help it settle.*

How to Use this Book

This book comprises three sections. The first part is an introduction to the history, preparation, and uses of the essences, and some of the theory that explains how they work. The main part of the book – the Materia Medica – is a compendium of the plants from which the principal essences are derived, with full details of the preparation and uses of each essence. The final section contains a series of highly informative indexes, allowing you to pinpoint suitable essences for your particular needs simply by looking up the key words that you would apply to your situation, such as the stage you are at in the cycle of life, your relationships with other people, or your emotional state.

BELOW **The Materia Medica, giving full details of the source plants and the essences, forms the heart of the book.**

BELOW **As well as the theory behind flower essences, the first part of the book includes full instructions on how to prepare your own essences at home.**

Step-by-step photography is used to explain the process.

A "signature box" contains details of each source plant's name, color, shape, and habitat.

Full details of the equipment that you will need are given.

Case studies illustrate some of the circumstances in which each essence can be beneficial.

Index entries consist of everyday terms that you might use to describe your own circumstances.

RIGHT **Indexes in the last part of the book provide a means of identifying the right essence to suit your emotional or relational state, and your time of life.**

The History of Flower Essences

ABORIGINAL PEOPLES *from all over the world have long used flowers in their rituals and ceremonies, aware of their subtle healing properties. Flower essence therapy as we know it today started in 1928 when Dr. Edward Bach began his work but is based on thousands of years of dependency on the plant kingdom for life itself.*

LEFT *An early apothecary making medicines.*

THE DOCTRINE OF CORRESPONDENCE

The physicians of Paracelsus' time believed that there were archetypes behind the material world to which material things corresponded. These basic archetypes were seen as the templates for every part of creation, and so there were correspondences between plants and animals, animals and humans, chemicals and organs, and so on. If a part of the body was sick, then the physician would turn to the corresponding archetype.

THE DOCTRINE OF SIGNATURES

As a graphologist might read your character from your handwriting, so would the physician be able to read the character of a plant from its color, smell, and how it grew. This would indicate how it was to be used as medicine, for example, chamomile has a center like a child's stomach, so this would be its area of influence. Investigation has shown that the active oils of chamomile are sedative to the nervous system, especially for children.

The way in which the plant grew was also significant. The fact that comfrey's leaf and stem fuse together suggested that it could cause broken bones to grow together. It was known as "knit-bone" and has been used for centuries to do just that. Comfrey ointment is still used today and druggists have isolated its gluey chemical – allontin.

Paracelsus' main premise was that all disease originated from our departure from our essential spiritual nature, due to the corruptibility of the mind and senses. Finding the right remedy would put us back in touch with the spirit within us, which alone is the true healer. What is important is that what he believed in worked. At that time he was famous, not so much for his own philosophy but for his practical and truly amazing cures.

METAMORPHOSIS

Goethe saw that underlying the myriad forms of plant life is the leaf. This archetypal shape of nature is acted upon by cosmic forces that produce root, stem, flower, and fruit. This metamorphosis, or power to transmute, is the key to the individuality of each particular plant and to its healing ability.

1493–1542	1749–1832	1755–1843
PARACELSUS Believed that the material universe could not be separated from the spiritual and that everything in creation was important. 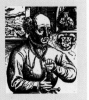	JOHANN WOLFGANG VON GOETHE Investigated the unique spiritual nature of each plant through observation of its growth. 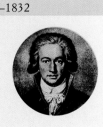	SAMUEL HAHNEMANN Pioneered remedies from nature, treating the whole person – body, mind, and spirit; developed the principles of homeopathy. 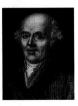

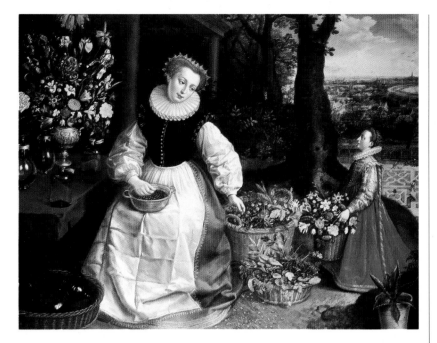

ABOVE *Flower essence therapy has a long tradition throughout history.*

He observed nature accurately, combining this with a close observation of his own responses. In this way he married scientific and artistic methods, and thus came to understand the spiritual identity of the plant – a practice that many flower essence-makers use today.

DR. EDWARD BACH
1886–1936

Bach was the first modern holistic healer to teach about the spiritual and emotional healing power of plants. Even as a boy he had an intense desire to find a simple,

natural method of healing that could be made and used by people themselves. He was strongly influenced by Samuel Hahnemann and Paracelsus. He was also probably affected by the lively development of esoteric studies of his time and was known to be an active member of the Masonic lodge. He initially studied medicine and homeopathy but in 1928 began creating flower essences. He moved from London to Wales where he discovered the method and preparation of flowers and spring water known as the 38 Bach Flower Remedies.

FLOWER ESSENCES IN THE 1970s

Although Bach felt he had made a complete system, it is obvious that other countries also have wonderful indigenous flowers that could be used as flower essences. So, in an unspoiled location in California, Richard Katz made the California Poppy into an essence. The flower is like a beautiful golden yellow cup that deepens into a rich orange toward the center.

In the 1970s, when this flower essence was made, California was the center of frenzied experimentation with hallucinogenic drugs. This essence reminds us that "true gold lies in the heart" rather than in the development of psychic powers.

In 1980 Patricia Kaminski began to codirect the Flower Essence Society, which has influenced others all over the world. Their repertory has grown from the original 38 essences to 103 and many more plants are being researched. The Flower Essence Society has set up a computer database that for over a decade has sifted and sorted a large amount of feedback from flower essence practitioners and clients.

1861–1925	1886–1936	1970
RUDOLPH STEINER Continued Goethe's work; believed in the power of feeling and observation and the need to be in touch with the unseen forces of nature. 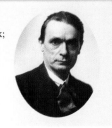	EDWARD BACH Influenced by the ideas of Hahnemann and Paracelsus, Bach created the first flower remedies.	FLOWER ESSENCE SOCIETY Influenced by Goethe, Steiner, and Dr. Edward Bach, F. E. S. experimented with making essences from Californian plants.

The Bach Flower Remedies

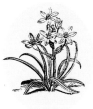

ABOVE *Star of Bethlehem, one of Bach's 38 remedies.*

DR.EDWARD BACH *created 38 flower essences. He divided his remedies into seven categories to describe the major positive qualities that he saw in humanity – the ability to be self-reliant, to lead and inspire others, to be alive to learning from each moment, to love and serve others, to be in charge of our own destinies, and to confront fear with faith and courage. The 38 essences that he made have enabled millions of sick people to regain their unique, positive potentials.*

Dr. Edward Bach studied medicine before joining University College, London, as a bacteriologist in 1913. Here, influenced by homeopathy, Bach developed vaccines from intestinal bacteria that cleansed the systems of the poisons that caused chronic disease. In 1919 he was offered a position at the London Homeopathic Hospital. Despite the fact that he was considered a medical genius by all who knew him, Bach remained unsatisfied. He wanted to use herbs rather than bacteria in his treatments and he was determined to carry further the homeopathic principle of treating the person and not the disease.

In 1928 he gave up his practice in London's Harley Street and went to Wales where he discovered the sun method of preparing flowers, which would be crucial to the development of his new system. His sensitivity to nature was such that he might hold a bloom in his hand and instinctively know which emotional state that flower would heal. Alternatively he would feel a negative mood overcome him only to find the positive solution in the discovery of his next remedy.

He observed that the morning plant dew contained potentized healing virtues of the whole plant. It was impractical to use this for large dosages so he developed his sun method of preparation and later his boiling method. He had made 12 remedies by the winter of 1932 and in 1935, over a year before his death, he had made another 26 remedies and Rescue Remedy, the composite flower essence made up of five Bach Remedies: Rock Rose, Impatiens, Star of Bethlehem, Clematis, and Cherry Plum. This remedy is often known as the 39th Remedy and is regarded as the most reliable remedy for shock and trauma (*see Combining and Combinations pp.124–5*).

Bach believed that true healing comes through illness since it provides us with the opportunity for understanding our own natures; physical relief without self-learning is only temporary at best. He developed a unique system of healing that he, and many others since, consider complete. He managed to take homeopathy one step further by using only nonharmful plants, plants that he believed were divinely enriched with healing powers similar to beautiful music, "which brings us nearer to our souls." This is his heritage: a most profound yet simple method of connecting ourselves to the healing source deep within ourselves.

THE 38 BACH FLOWER REMEDIES

Bach organized the remedies in groups according to seven different character types. Each remedy is shown with the positive characteristics of their type first, and then the negative characteristics. These negative characteristics will dominate if the person is out of balance.

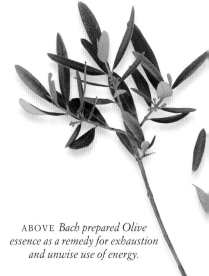

ABOVE *Bach prepared Olive essence as a remedy for exhaustion and unwise use of energy.*

THE 38 BACH FLOWER REMEDIES

PLANT	POSITIVE	NEGATIVE
REMEDIES FOR LONELINESS		
Heather	True interest and connection with others.	Self-centered; unable to relate to others.
Impatiens	Relaxation; cooperation; balanced poise.	Impatience leading to physical, emotional, or mental tension.
Water Violet	Approachable; connected to others.	Overly self-reliant; sense of superiority.
REMEDIES FOR OVERCARE FOR THE WELFARE OF OTHERS		
Beech	See that the world is good.	Over-meticulous, critical.
Chicory	Generous love.	Emotional neediness; manipulation; overattachment.
Rock Water, potentized spring water	Kind to oneself; open-minded.	Overly self-critical; has rigid beliefs.
Vervain	Self-containment and relaxation.	Overenergetic enthusiasm and idealism.
Vine	Desire to give genuine service to others.	Domineering or controlling.
REMEDIES FOR LACK OF INTEREST IN PRESENT CIRCUMSTANCES		
Chestnut Bud	Is able to learn from experience.	Makes the same mistakes again and again.
Clematis	Alert; grounded; able to realize vision.	Daydreamer; ungrounded; impractical.
Honeysuckle	Able to find joy in the present.	Caught up in the past.
Mustard	Understands reason for moodiness; cheerful.	Gloomy, depressed feelings for no known reason.
Olive	Spiritual renewal; proper use of energy.	For exhaustion; depletion; unwise use of energy.
White Chestnut	Uncluttered mind; peace.	For people whose thoughts constantly spin.
Wild Rose	Enthusiasm; purposefulness.	For resignation; apathy.
REMEDIES FOR THOSE OVERSENSITIVE TO INFLUENCES AND IDEAS		
Agrimony	Honesty toward self and others; inner peace.	For those who hide their feelings behind a happy face.
Centaury	Balanced service and trueness to own needs.	For people who serve others to their own cost.
Holly	Love; humility; tolerance.	For jealousy; hatred; suspicion.
Walnut	Skillful change toward new and true goals.	For stressful change and major life transitions.
REMEDIES FOR UNCERTAINTY		
Cerato	Wise discrimination; self-reliance.	Lack of trust in own wisdom.
Gentian	Revives courage and strength.	Becomes discouraged by setbacks.
Gorse	Sees hope.	Feels that it is pointless to try.
Hornbeam	Strengthens belief in the ability to cope.	Finds it hard to face the day's work
Scleranthus	Clear, balanced overview.	Indecisiveness and an inability to choose between alternatives.
Wild Oat	Clarity of purpose; contentment.	Confusion about one's direction in life.
REMEDIES FOR FEAR		
Aspen	Grounded in oneself; trusting in the unknown.	Vague fears of unknown things.
Cherry Plum	Trust in higher benevolent power.	Fear of losing self-control, giving way to harmful impulses.
Mimulus	Faces up to things bravely.	Nervous, shy, and afraid of known things.
Red Chestnut	Can keep a boundary between self and others.	Overanxious about the welfare of others.
Rock Rose	Courage, peace, and mental clarity	Terror and panic.
REMEDIES FOR DESPONDENCY AND DESPAIR		
Crab Apple	Cleansing, inner purity, spiritual evolution.	Feeling unclean or impure.
Elm	Strengthens the ability to carry on.	For people who become overwhelmed temporarily.
Larch	Self-confident; self-expressive.	For lack of confidence to try.
Oak	Flexible strength; support for oneself.	For exhausted people who struggle on.
Pine	Sense of proportion; release of self-blame.	For people who feel guilty for everything.
Star of Bethlehem	Peace; tranquillity; soothing.	For shock; trauma.
Sweet Chestnut	Restoration of faith in life and in self.	For deepest despair; complete anguish.
Willow	Self-responsibility; acceptance.	Bitterness and resentment; feelings of victimization.

CHICORY

WILD ROSE

The Aura

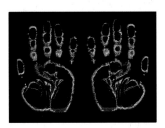

ABOVE *The aura that surrounds a person reveals his or her physical and mental well-being.*

MANY SCIENTISTS *are turning for inspiration to the mystics to help them resolve the mysteries of creation. They too are coming to the conclusion that the human body, like everything else in the universe, is made from light and sound. Halos painted around the saints show their perfect connection with this light energy. We lesser mortals too have auras, which, to those who can see, give us information that is as unique as our fingerprints.*

THE AURA AND THE ENERGETIC SYSTEM OF THE BODY

The aura is often described as an energy envelope that surrounds a person's body. It continually changes color and shape as it interacts with other energies in the environment. Until recently only clairvoyants could see the colors and shapes that surround our body and that are created by our fluctuating moods. However, in the 1960s Russians Semyon and Valentina Kirlian developed a form of photography that could detect the life-force energy field surrounding plants, crystals, animals, and human beings. They showed that even when a leaf is torn, it still has a complete shape in its energy field. From this they deduced that there was an organizing intelligence in the plant. Kirlian photography has been useful in showing the energy impact on our bodies of, for example, spiritual healing, wholesome food, and flower essences. A person in good health will emit strong radiations, while a person in poor health will emit weak radiations.

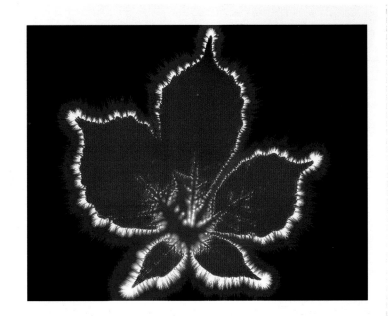

ABOVE *This Kirlian picture detects the energy surrounding a chestnut leaf.*

This breakthrough in detecting energy fields was developed further by Harry Oldfield who makes videotapes of the human auric field. These tapes can be interpreted to show the cause of physical problems. Expert analysis can also point out how the brown smudges and gray leaks that appear instead of the rainbow colors of good health are potential causes of problems in the physical body. Skillfully interpreted by an expert in the field, these videotapes can demonstrate how the vibrational healing of crystals and flower essences change the auric field to bring back rainbow colors, thus healing our energy field and inhibiting further negative conditions that cause ill-health.

THE HEALING POWER OF COLOR

Each color in the aura is created by the whirling energy centers, or "chakras," that are situated along the spine. When we are feeling hale and hearty we have a radiant rainbow body, and when we are not, we are like the sky in bad weather, clouded over.

People have always been instinctively aware of the healing power of color. So not surprisingly color is an extremely important part of the signature of a flower. You may have noticed how you tend to wear clothes that are the right color to suit or alter your mood or emotion. In the same way, pink flowers will soften our hearts, and yellow flowers, like the sun, will cheer us up. But with flower essences, the shape and growth habits of the

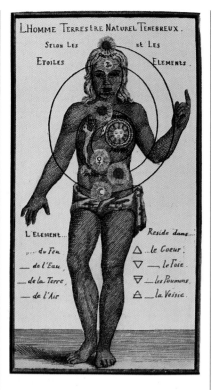

ABOVE *The colors of the aura are created by the body's energy centers, known as chakras.*

particular plant we are using also bring their influence to bear on our bodies' energy systems.

The glorious color of flowers not only attracts insects as pollinators but also indicates to the flower essence-maker which of the five subtle elements the plant is transforming. These elements are present throughout the whole of creation and are embodied in the human form in the chakra system. So, for example, when red predominates it is increasing fire energy; when blue predominates it is working with cooling, contracting energies, and so on. So the color signals to us what energy that plant is working with. Just as there is a multitude of different colors and hues in the blooms, so there is a multitude of different ways in which the plants work with energies.

COLORS THAT HEAL

WHITE ❀ helps you to connect to your own purity and to others in a spiritual way.

MAGENTA ❀ is the color of the purest spiritual energy. It can help you to let go of old feelings that inhibit change.

VIOLET ❀ encourages self-respect and dignity, and can help you connect with your true sense of identity.

BLUE ❀ promotes peace, calm, and consideration. Too little blue and you tend to be scattered and inconsistent, too much and you may be depressed.

GREEN ❀ stands in the middle of the spectrum between blue and yellow, and is associated with the heart and with harmony and balance.

ROSE PINKS ❀ are also connected with the heart. They help in our emotional development, bringing active love for the self and others.

YELLOW ❀ encourages detached cheerfulness. Too much yellow may lead to self-criticism, not enough may make you critical of others.

ORANGE ❀ represents the power of deep emotion, enabling enjoyment of sensual contact and dance, and appreciation of life.

RED ❀ increases energy and alertness. Too much can mean an excess of heat and anger; too little indicates insufficient energy to think clearly.

MAROON ❀ helps you to bring your energy and your will together.

There are now many forms of diagnosis that use color not only to detect passing moods but also to detect deeper problems that exist in the systems of the body. One of these is the Luscher color test, which may help you with your self-diagnosis.

How Flower Essences Work

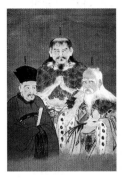

LEFT *The* Emperor's Classic *states that negative emotions affect our life energy.*

PLANTS IN THE WILD *must have mastered their environment to survive. The essence is made from the plant when it is flowering and at the height of its power. The bloom conveys its healthy qualities into water, aided by the magnetic energy of the sun. When we make a good match to our mood pattern, these qualities boost our vitality and give us greater strength to master our own environment.*

PREVENTION IS BETTER THAN CURE

It has long been known that to treat and cure disease it is necessary to search out its origins. In one of the most important texts of Chinese medicine, *The Yellow Emperor's Classic of Internal Medicine*, it states clearly that negative emotions affect the way that life energy circulates in the body: excess "joy injures the heart, anger injures the liver, over-concentration injures the spleen, anxiety injures the lungs, fear injures the kidneys." In more recent times biochemical research has shown that chronic feeling states such as anger or shame produce permanent changes in endocrine chemistry. The long-term effect of suppressed anger, for instance, may send the blood pressure up. This is understood in general terms as stress. Stress may be imprinted on the physical body, in the same way as music is imprinted on a compact disk.

Psychosomatic illness results from biochemical changes caused by the intensification or suppression of the very feelings mentioned long ago in the *Emperor's Classic.* Positive feelings also have a direct impact on the immune system in a positive way. In other words, you can "head off" many physical problems, both chronic and acute, by deciding for yourself in what way your feelings and attitudes could be weakening your resistance to disease. So in flower essence therapy we are attempting to focus much more on creating health, rather than treating sickness, using the flower essences as catalysts for awareness.

FLOWER ESSENCE THERAPY

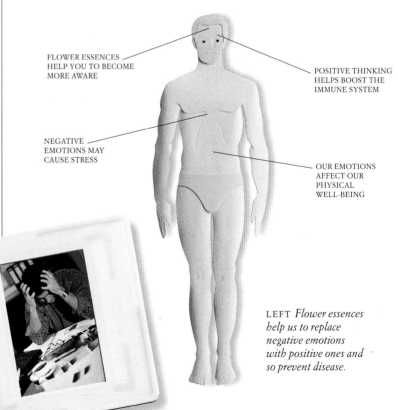

FLOWER ESSENCES HELP YOU TO BECOME MORE AWARE

POSITIVE THINKING HELPS BOOST THE IMMUNE SYSTEM

NEGATIVE EMOTIONS MAY CAUSE STRESS

OUR EMOTIONS AFFECT OUR PHYSICAL WELL-BEING

RIGHT *Stress, often caused by suppressed emotions, may cause a rise in blood pressure.*

LEFT *Flower essences help us to replace negative emotions with positive ones and so prevent disease.*

HOW DOES A FLOWER ESSENCE WORK?

We are still learning just how a little flower can uplift us or help us to study more efficiently. Recent research has shown that water has a "memory." It therefore seems that in flower essence therapy an imprint of the flower's properties is held in the water that contained it and is then transferred to us.

Another important concept in vibrational medicine is that of resonance. If you put several violins in a room and draw a string across one of them, then the others will make a matching sound. So the microdose of the flower imprint resonates throughout your energy system, gradually permeating your aura with color, light, and even sound.

Sages have for millennia maintained that each human being is a microcosm of the macrocosm. So the influences that have made the flower also influence us. The energetic quality of a flower amplifies that potential within us and brings out our better qualities.

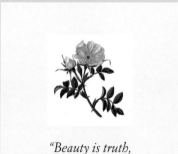

*"Beauty is truth,
truth beauty, –
that is all
Ye know on earth and all
ye need to know."*

JOHN KEATS

HOW TO KNOW IF THE ESSENCE IS WORKING

In the case studies in the following section the word "realization" is frequently used. Often the major effect of an essence is to heighten our understanding of what might be wrong with us.

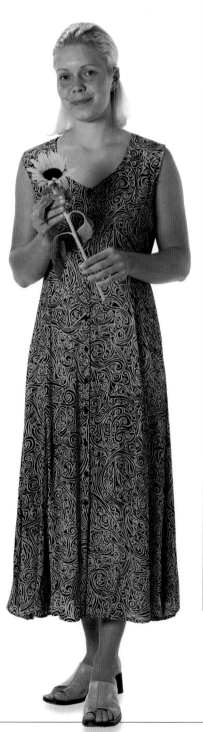

This understanding arises as a result of an increased vitality in the subtle body and might be experienced as a sudden feeling of relief or joy or a movement toward emotional expression. For example, after using Dandelion essence, one woman reported that she found herself swinging her hips as she carried her basketful of shopping. She had never done that before. The freeing quality of the essence gave her a new sense of her body and the rhythm inherent in it. Bach describes the effect of an essence as being like beautiful music that uplifts the spirit. It is important to take note of these small signs and acknowledge them. Like a small child doing a difficult task, our often very fragile movements toward good health need a lot of encouragement.

However grownup and responsible we are in our society and to our family, most of us are spiritually immature. This makes us all equal, however much money we have and whatever our role in life. The message of the flowers is always utterly humanitarian and spiritual. It is about finding our place within the whole of creation, not grabbing a little part of it and dominating it for our own purposes. Flower essences have a truly ecological message, since they always speak from their own nature about the mystery and beauty inherent in the heart of creation itself. We have much to learn from them.

LEFT *Flower essences will
have a positive effect on you,
both physically and mentally,
and help you to feel revitalized.*

Making Your Own Essences

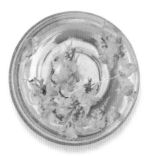

A FLOWER ESSENCE *is the fleeting energy of the bloom, the plant's unique expression preserved, using the elements of nature: earth, air, fire, and water. There is also, of course, the important fifth element – spirit.*

LEFT *Pick only fresh, vital-looking blossoms to make your essence.*

You can enhance this fifth element through your own sensitivity to nature's generosity, so only pick wild flowers where there are large groups.

The growth of the flower is dependent upon the right balance of the four elements – good earth, air, fire (sun), and water. Most essences are made using the power of the sun so you need plenty of sunshine. You also need to feel focused and aware of yourself so that you know which plant attracts you. Prepare yourself to be sensitive and receptive so that you can connect with nature. Find a calm, unpolluted place in which to make the essence – no overhead cables, no agricultural sprays of any sort, no car fumes.

Remember that the water in which you collect the essence of the flower, the mother tincture, need only be a small amount. Half a pint of mother tincture could eventually make 648,000 dosage bottles. So stay small, unless you decide to use the mother tinctures regularly in baths.

THE FIFTH ELEMENT

The most important factor in making a flower essence is your personal relationship with the plant itself. Most essence-makers say that the plant chooses them and asks to be made into an essence. If you don't feel this immediate sense of

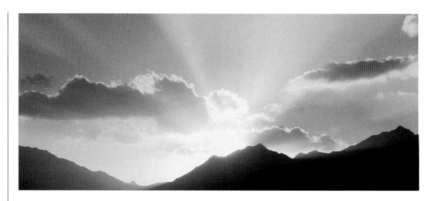

ABOVE *The best time to make your essences is at dawn when everything is fresh.*

connection and you still want to make an essence, then spend time getting to know the plant. Study it. Sit quietly with the flower, and maybe draw it. You may even want to read about its botany, history, or folklore. This is a sign of respect to the plant, like finding out about a new friend.

Only ever make one essence at a time. Through your sensitivity you are making your own magic. The more mechanically you do it, the less potency your essence will have. Early in the morning, at dawn if you can, go and sit with your plant until you feel the right time has come for making your essence. Then give thanks to nature and to the plant itself for this opportunity to tap its wonderful healing powers.

EQUIPMENT

You will need the following items of equipment:
- a small clean glass bowl
- a bottle in which to mix the brandy and flower-charged water
- good fresh water (If there is a clear spring nearby, that is ideal. Or if you can, collect rainwater. Otherwise use a local bottled water. Bottled spring water is fine if you can't get any of these.)
- a good fruit brandy, organic if possible – if not, the best you can afford to buy
- a funnel for pouring the mother tincture into a bottle

THE SUN METHOD

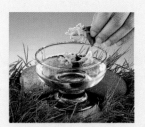 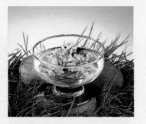 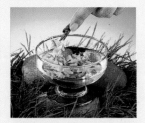 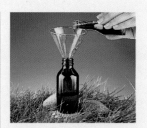

1 *Pick some of the most vital-looking blossoms from separate plants and place them in a bowl that has been nearly filled with spring water. To avoid touching the blooms with your hand, use a leaf to carry them.*

2 *Completely cover the surface of the water with the flowers.*
   Leave the bowl in the sunshine for around three hours, near other plants, with as little shadow falling on it as possible.

3 *Check the blooms from time to time to see if they are looking limp. If so, it generally means that their vital force has gone into the water. If you do not have continuous sunshine for three hours, decide whether or not you want to carry on. You may want to start again another day. Use your intuition about this. Lift the blooms out of the water with a twig or leaf.*

4 *Pour your essence into a clean, empty bottle with an equal amount of brandy. This is your mother tincture. Be sure to label it clearly.*
   If you have too much essence water, then pour it back onto the earth under the plant and give thanks.

THE BOILING METHOD

Many flowering trees need some extra fire energy to bring out their essential qualities, especially if they blossom in dull weather. This energy can be added to the essence by using the boiling method of preparation. Bach's Walnut remedy is made by the boiling method.

Additional equipment
As well as the basic equipment listed above, you will need an enamel or stainless steel pan (enamel is best – don't use aluminum; it will contaminate the water), filter paper for straining the debris, and some method of heating.

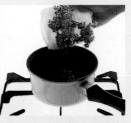 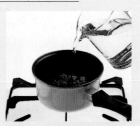 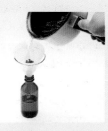

1 *Instead of picking only the blossoms, include some of the twigs. Put them in the bottom of your pan.*

Other methods
These include Judy Griffin's cold infusion and extraction process and Andreas Korte's crystal method.

2 *Ideally cover them with spring water and immediately put the pan on to boil. If this is not possible, cover the pan, take it straight home and put it on to boil as soon as you get in. Leave it to simmer for 30 minutes, using another twig to keep the blossoms and twigs under the water. Leave the pan outside to cool.*

3 *Carefully remove the twigs and blossoms with another twig and filter the essence into a bottle with an equal amount of brandy. Label the mother tincture clearly.*

Using Your Flower Essences

FLOWER ESSENCES *are simple to use and can easily complement many other therapies. They will not counteract, or be counteracted by ordinary medicines prescribed by your physician. This makes them an invaluable adjunct to any health plan. Flower essences can be used with any other form of healing because, unlike homeopathic medicines, they cannot be antidoted by other substances.*

Stock is prepared by putting two drops of the mother tincture into a 1 fl. oz (30ml) bottle filled with pure brandy. Stock essences are also available commercially. There are several other easy ways of using the stock essence.

• You can dilute the stock directly into a glass of water, and sip it at intervals during the day. Keep the mixture clean by placing a lid over the glass. Stir it with a twig from the same plant or any clean implement in order to "wake it up" before you drink it.

• Add about 20 drops of stock essence into a normal-sized bathtub of warm water. You can use your favorite bath additives too, but don't overdo it. Stir the water in a figure-of-eight motion for at least one minute to help the essences spread in the water. Soak for about 20 minutes. Wrap yourself in a bathrobe and then rest for at least another 20 minutes.

• Some essences are effective when they are rubbed directly onto the skin. They can be used as part of massage with oils, acupressure, and polarity therapy. (*See the supportive technique for each flower in the Materia Medica, pp. 22–119*).

DOSAGE BOTTLES

You can usually buy glass dosage bottles from a druggist or from your essence supplier, if there is one near you. Use a 1fl. oz (30ml) bottle with a dropper then make up the dosage bottle as follows.

• If you live in a hot climate fill the bottle with brandy to between one eighth and one quarter, then top it up with water. (If you are alcohol-sensitive you can use vegetable glycerine or cider vinegar.) Alternatively keep your bottle in the refrigerator. Nearly fill the bottle with spring water or the best water you have.

• Add two to four drops from the stock essence.

• Before use, rhythmically shake or lightly tap the bottle to energize it.

• Place four drops under your tongue, or in a small amount of water. Don't let the dropper touch your mouth otherwise it will pick up bacteria, which will sour the flower essence.

• You can reuse your dosage bottle and pipette by boiling them in water for ten minutes and drying

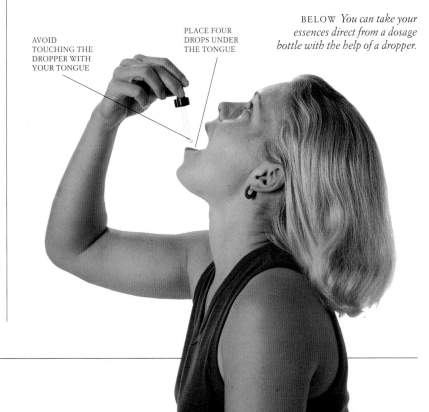

AVOID TOUCHING THE DROPPER WITH YOUR TONGUE

PLACE FOUR DROPS UNDER THE TONGUE

BELOW *You can take your essences direct from a dosage bottle with the help of a dropper.*

them upside down. With care you can wash and reuse the rubber caps too.

• You can add some drops from your dosage bottle to half a glass of water, and by stirring it first one way and then the other you can bring the essence alive. Sip it slowly. It is also possible to add the essence to fruit juices or spring water. Normally you would take your remedy four times a day. A dosage bottle will usually last you about three weeks.

It is important to note that potency is increased not by taking more of an essence at one time, but by increasing the frequency of use during emergency or acute situations. Once you have what you believe is the right essence for you, it is important to use it with patience and consistency. You may at some time have an awareness crisis, or what you could call a mental aggravation. This is because the holistic nature of the essence can bring up feelings you may not have acknowledged in the past. This can be uncomfortable. If you can, talk to a friend or therapist about your feelings. If this does not help, then reduce the dose, or change your remedy to counteract your difficulty. Children or highly sensitive people may need to decrease the frequency of use. For some very sensitive people even using one dose once a week can be enough.

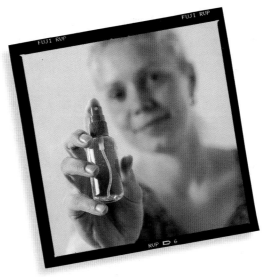

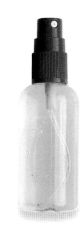

ABOVE AND LEFT *Enhance the environment by using flower essences in a spray to clean the atmosphere.*

SPRAY BOTTLE

A commercially bought vaporizer or spray bottle can be made up in the same way as a dosage bottle. Spray the mixture onto your body and in the air around you.

CREAMS, OILS, AND LOTIONS

These can be made up by adding six to ten drops from the stock of each essence to 1oz. (30gm) of cream, oil, or lotion. You can use these in addition to, or instead of, taking the flower essence orally.

COMPRESSES

Compresses are very useful for dealing with intense pains or persistent problems. Put two drops of essence in half a glass of water and soak a piece of cloth in it. Put it on the appropriate part of the body and leave it for approximately ten minutes.

SOAK THE COMPRESS IN WATER WITH TWO DROPS OF FLOWER ESSENCE BEFORE USE

APPLY COLD COMPRESS TO THE PROBLEM AREA

RIGHT *Cold compresses may be applied directly to the skin to provide instant relief from intense pain.*

The Materia Medica

THE 48 PLANTS *and one sea creature described in this section have been used to make flower essences because of their powerful ability to help with mental, emotional, and spiritual difficulties. One of the reasons these particular essences have been chosen is for the range of problems for which they can be used. The plants here come from all corners of the world. Some common wild plants have been selected by a number of essence-makers, drawn to them because of the plants' established place in folklore and herbalism. Others have been introduced as medicines only recently.*

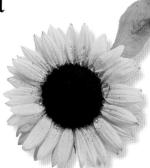

ABOVE *Flowers, such as the majestic sunflower, have wonderful healing properties and can help many ailments.*

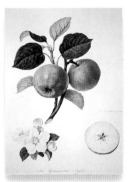

ABOVE *Many of the plants used in flower essence therapy, such as apple, have a long history of use in herbalism.*

Although flower essences are effective, they are completely harmless and nonaddictive. You can regulate your dosage so that you are totally in control of the essence's potency. There are no rules about when you can or cannot use a flower essence. Even if you are feeling fine, you can still use flower essences to help you feel even better. Once you've tried them and felt their beneficial effects, you will never want to be without your essences.

It is possible for you to use the flower essences yourself to help you solve your own problems and develop your true potential. One of the aims of this section is to support you in this, or at least to help you get started. However, interdependency is a key concept in the natural world, so join with others and share your quest, if and when you can. The unfolding of our deeper selves is generally easier and more rewarding done with the support of our friends, family, or therapist.

LEFT *With help from the Materia Medica, you can begin to use the essences yourself.*

How to Use the Materia Medica

The Materia Medica provides a comprehensive compendium of the plants from which the essences are derived. They are presented in alphabetical order by their botanical names, but if you know only the common name of a particular plant, the index will guide you to the right entry. The information for each plant is presented in a form that is easy to use and follow. After a general introduction, the signature box gives alternative names for the plant and a detailed description of the plant's appearance and its habitat and growth pattern. There is also information about the folklore concerning the plant and its usage. A notes box details the plant's therapeutic actions, how the essence is made, and how it can be combined with other essences. For each plant, there is also a case history describing the beneficial effect of the essence in practice.

Introduction
Each spread has a general botanical introduction to the plant, providing an overview of its characteristics and family.

Case study
This is taken from genuine therapeutic experience with the essences. Details have been changed for the sake of confidentiality, but the essential qualities of the case have been retained.

Notes
A paragraph on therapeutic actions summarizes the plant's potential action. A method of making is suggested for each flower. Additional techniques and therapies are also mentioned.

Signature
Both the scientific name and any common names are explained here. This section attempts to summarize in words what the plant symbolizes in its color, shape, habitat, and growth patterns. Its name and usage are also covered to capture the overall message of the plant.

Ways of using and use in combination
Suggestions are given for other essences that can be used effectively in a combination, but check to see what is appropriate. Use your own discretion.

Key words
These are to help you get an idea of the areas in which the flower essence can help. These words do not cover all of the possibilities. You will find out more about the overall nature of the healing energy of the flower by reading about its signature.

Folklore and usage
This section details the historical beliefs, myths, and usage of the flower.

Affirmation
This is related to the signature of the plant and its proven use in healing. The affirmation helps to direct your thoughts and support the flower's healing power.

Challenge
This is to help you focus on the healing energy of the flower. This challenge is derived from a study of the flower's signature, what essence-makers say about it, and case histories.

ABOVE **The flower essences in this section are each organized in a similar way for ease of reference.**

Achillea millefolium

Yarrow

Y ARROW *is an important member of the Asteraceae or aster branch of the Compositae (daisy) family. It is often categorized as a kind of sneezewort with chamomile, mayweed, and corn marigold. There are about 100 different species that grow mainly in temperate regions of the world. Yarrow is a hardy perennial herb and grows prolifically in grass, meadows, lawns, waste places, pastures, and by the roadside.*

RIGHT *Growing up to 3ft. (1m) high, the yarrow is a hardy perennial herb that thrives in sunny conditions.*

SIGNATURE

& *A protective umbrella filters out harm* &

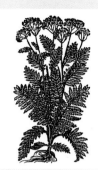

ACHILLEA MILLEFOLIUM

Name

Other names for yarrow include carpenter's wort, staunch weed, milfoil, nosebleed, and thousand weed. Its Latin name derives from Achilles, the Greek warrior, and *millefolium*, a thousand leaves, because of its much divided leaves. Achilles healed the wounded warrior Telephus with yarrow.

It is called carpenter's wort by the French because of its supposed ability to heal wounds made by carpenters' tools.

Color/shape

The white flowers are individually so small they might be mistaken as coming from the *Umbelliferae* family. The stems are stiff, furrowed, and woolly, and branch to create a cluster of flowerheads that function as a single large flower, like an umbrella. This radiant white protective shield looks as though it can filter out and deflect anything harmful that might be present in the environment.

Yarrow's leaf is particularly beautiful. It has one lone midrib, which is feathered twice in two divisions of long pointed segments, each bearing almost 1,000 little leaves.

This is where its name milfoil originated.

These multiple indentations of the leaf can be seen as a metaphor for the way in which we can be sensitive to the environment in 1,000 ways. Sensitivity to the environment is very useful, especially if we need to respond to others in a healing way, but it needs to be combined with strength.

Habitat and growth pattern

The yarrow has deep water-gathering tap roots that make it a very tough plant. It is a natural survivor, coping with even the lawnmower; it usually flowers after the first cut, keeping just below the level of most blades. It thrives by the sides of roads even in polluted traffic. Yarrow is a strong survivor that can in turn support our ability to thrive in circumstances that may be threatening.

Key words

POSITIVE: *Strengthening of aura, appropriately sensitive, strong immune system.*
NEGATIVE: *Immune disturbances, vulnerability to emotional and psychic toxicity, oversensitivity to environmental influences.*

Challenge

To stand protected and healed, ready to respond sensitively to others.

RIGHT *Legend says that yarrow was placed in the hands of the infant Jesus as he lay in the manger.*

FOLKLORE AND USAGE

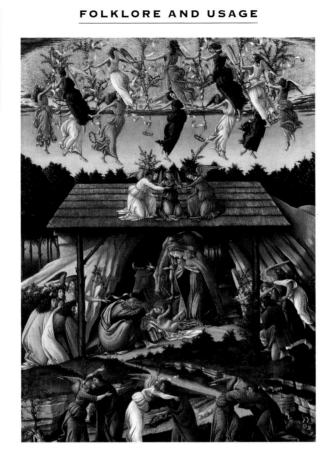

NOTES

Therapeutic actions
Yarrow gives integrity and strength to the aura so that we can maintain awareness of the suffering of others without being overwhelmed, and be protected from environmental pollution.

Method of making essence
Sun method. Be sure to use only plants that grow in environmentally perfect conditions, in a place away from pollution and overhead cables.

Ways of using and use in combination
Use in dosage bottle with Self-heal and Walnut, or Garlic; use in a spray around the room; rub a little diluted stock essence into your hands and give yourself an auric massage by circulating your hands all round your body; use with Yarrow Special Formula, (see p.125).

Best supportive technique
Exercises with sound such as polarity therapy exercises; aromatherapy.

✤ Yarrow was reportedly the first herb placed in the baby Jesus' hand, perhaps to signal both his healing powers and vulnerability.

✤ The yarrow plant has long been associated with the healing of wounds and the stemming of blood flow.

✤ Externally it is used to treat slow-healing wounds, skin rashes, eczema, and chapped skin, and for opening the pores of the skin to create an artificial fever to release toxins from the body.

✤ The skin is the body's major organ of defense and elimination. It also literally holds us together. Yarrow does this on an auric level.

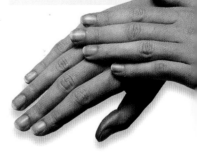

ABOVE *Yarrow essence can be applied directly to the skin to treat complaints such as eczema and chapped skin.*

Allium sativum

Garlic

GARLIC *originated in India or central Asia and was introduced into Britain by the Romans who used it in their medicine.*

The Allium *belongs to the Lily family. This is one of the largest families of flowering plants, and certainly one of the most important horticulturally. It includes the lilies and numerous other outstandingly beautiful cultivated flowers, for example, tulips and hyacinths, and also vegetables such as onions, leeks, and asparagus.*

The members of the Lily family all have juicy bulbs or rhizomes stored with food. They are connected with the feminine ability to hold nourishment. Garlic is the fieriest of all these gentle bulbs.

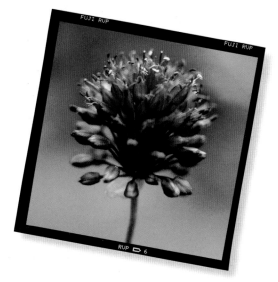

ABOVE *The garlic species has purplish-white flowers that grow in spherical clusters at the end of a long, straight stem.*

SIGNATURE

❧ *Fiery power combats all fears* ☙

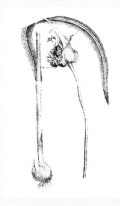

ALLIUM SATIVUM

Name
Garlic is also called stinkweed, gypsies' onions, poor man's treacle. Treacle was used as a blood cleanser in folk medicine until the mid-20th century, but if you couldn't afford to use it, garlic was used instead, hence poor man's treacle.

The word garlic comes from the Anglo-Saxon *garleac* – *gar* **for spear and** *leac* **meaning leak. The long pointed leaves look like spears pointing skyward. Its Latin name** *Allium* **is from** *celtical*, **which means caustic, a reference to the strong taste, and** *sativa* **meaning planted deliberately.**

Color/shape
The purplish-white flowers are in spherical clusters at the end of stalks that grow directly out of the bulbs. It is like a globe of purifying white, tinged with ethereal strength.

The bulb is covered with a purplish skin, so it is clear that some properties of the bulb are channeled through the hollow tube of the stem into the flower itself.

This ability to penetrate is important since it enables the garlic to permeate the body and remove deep pockets of infection. The flower has a similar impact on the psyche, penetrating and removing the hidden fears that cause putrefaction of the psyche.

Habitat and growth pattern
When cut, garlic is highly aromatic with a very fiery taste. In the soil the bulb has a purple-reddish skin that reflects its grounded power. It obviously has tremendous power to repel invaders particularly insects, such as aphids, by creating a strong boundary around itself.

CASE STUDY

Marjorie, a 40–year-old, had to give a presentation to her work colleagues.
She was very nervous indeed. Although three months away, just thinking about it overwhelmed her with fear. She had no idea what she was frightened of, but her solar plexus felt so tight that it was even difficult to breathe. She had suffered from candidiasis for a long time and that was getting worse too.

Marjorie was advised to take a Garlic essence bath regularly and within two weeks she reported feeling a lot better. She started to remember incidents in her childhood when she would be completely overwhelmed by fear of her mother and unable to stand up for herself. She began to confront these feelings and came to a realistic awareness of what this new speaking role would entail. She stopped being paralyzed by fear and worked hard on writing her speech. She realized it was an ideal opportunity to tackle her standing in her profession and that in fact she was ready to move on to the next step in her career.

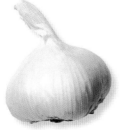

ABOVE *Garlic has many medicinal uses. It helps prevent colds, reduces blood pressure, and has antiseptic properties.*

FOLKLORE AND USAGE

❖ Garlic is one of the oldest medicinal remedies known to us. According to Islamic legend, garlic and onion grew up at Satan's feet after he stepped out of the Garden of Eden. The bulb consists of cloves grouped together that were thought to resemble the devil's cloven feet. Garlic was most famously used throughout Europe as a protection against vampires.

❖ Dr. Shook, the great American herbalist, said that he had seen it cure, among other things, "tuberculosis, asthma, bronchitis, several skin diseases, various ulcers." He used it as a paste applied to the soles of the feet, it was allowed to remain there to soak through the skin, fumigate the body, and heal purulent diseases. The Chinese used it as a treatment against leprosy.

❖ During World War I, garlic juice was used as an antiseptic on wounds. More recently it has been scientifically proved that its rich sulfur compounds are a digestive stimulant. It is antiseptic, assists circulation, and is useful for headaches.

BELOW *The Arabs believe that garlic grew at Satan's feet as he left the Garden of Eden.*

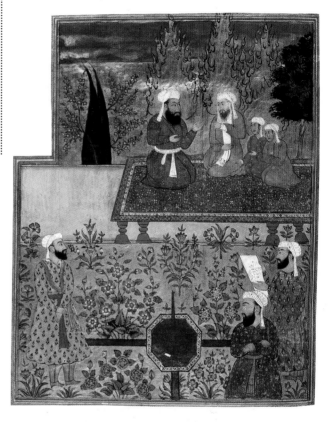

AFFIRMATION
My inner fire is overcoming all obstacles.

Key words
POSITIVE: *Courage, wholeness, resistance.*
NEGATIVE: *Fearful, weak, low vitality, viral infection.*

Challenge
To activate inner fire in order to take hold of life fully and combat fears.

NOTES

Therapeutic actions
A psychic antibiotic for overvulnerability to disease; helps to release deep insecurities and fears.

Method of making essence
Sun method.

Ways of using and use in combination
With Self-heal and Larch.

Best supportive technique
Simple assertiveness training.

Anthemis nobilis Chamaemelum nobile

Chamomile

ANTHEMIS *is a branch of the* Compositae *or daisy family. It belongs to the subdivision of* Asteracea*. There are about 100 species of them, including* asters *and* daisies *in the northern hemisphere,* brachycomes *and* oleria *in Australasia and* grindelia *and* solidagos *(golden rod) in North and South America. This species grows in western Europe, in southern England, Wales, and Ireland, usually in sandy soils, in grassy places, on heaths and commons, banks, and roadsides. It has not become naturalized in the United States. Chamomile tea is common to most of the world as an everyday drink to soothe stress and anxiety.*

BELOW *The center of the chamomile flower is domed, suggesting a raised stomach. This was taken as the signature of the plant.*

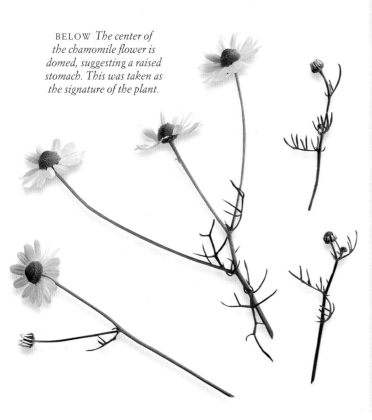

🌹 *Brings sunny calm to daily strife* 🌹

Name
This little flower is also called Roman chamomile because its use was common in Rome. *Anthemis* is a Greek word that signifies the flower kingdom itself. *Anthemis nobilis* is the usual term for chamomile in herbal and garden books, but in botanical literature *Chamaemelum nobile* is used. *Chamoemelon* is Greek for "earth apple," because of its delicate applelike fragrance.

Botanists find classifying many members of this family a frustrating process. This is in fact relevant to some of its signature, which is connected with getting upset over small things. Nature is infinite in its variety and, as the great scientist and poet Goethe pointed out, it is important to look at the relationship between plants to find meaning, not just to categorize.

Chamomile was called "patience in adversity" in the Victorian language of the flowers, and named as "the good, capped sister, with a thousand smiles" by the Belgian dramatist Maeterlinck.

Color/shape
Around midsummer, wild chamomile plants produce daisylike flowerheads, each one on a long stalk; 18 white rays emanate from a domed yellow center disk, suggesting the clarity of outgoing energy.

The rays droop as they age. The fruit is small and dry. As it forms, the hill of the center becomes increasingly conical, like an old person's stomach muscles relaxing.

Chamomile has stems that gently undulate and leaves that are finely divided into threadlike segments. This is reminiscent of the feathery appearance of branches of the nervous system. The whole plant is downy and gray-green in color, soothing, and easy on the eye.

Habitat and growth pattern
Chamomile has many creeping, rooting stems and pleasantly scented leaves that form a dense mat if left alone. It is wonderful to walk on because of the beautiful smell of the crushed leaves and flowers. It seems to thrive, even when flattened.

AFFIRMATION

I am resilient,
calm, and cheerful.

Key words

POSITIVE:
*Resilient,
sunny, calm.*
NEGATIVE:
*Downtrodden, moody,
nervous frustration.*

Challenge

*To be renewed every
day, like the sun,
with healing
and calm for the self
and for others.*

NOTES

Therapeutic actions
*Calms and soothes the
nerves; helps the release of
tension, anxiety, and fear;
supports deep relaxation;
helps to turn frustration
into acceptance.*

**Method of making
essence**
Sun method.

**Ways of using and
use in combination**
*Use in dosage bottle, or
as a massage oil over the
stomach at night; make a
cup of chamomile tea and
put a few drops of
chamomile essence in it
when you are feeling
overstressed; try combining
Chamomile with any of the
following: Self-heal,
Chicory, Valerian, Crowea,
or Garlic.*

Best supportive technique
*Make sure you relax in
some sunshine or good
light every day.*

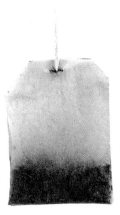

ABOVE *Chamomile tea
is recommended for
menstrual cramp and
as an aid to restful sleep.*

FOLKLORE AND USAGE

❁ The Egyptians consecrated chamomile to the sun god Ra and planted it on graves as a symbol that the deceased would be reborn, as the sun is reborn each morning.

❁ In 900 B.C. Asclepiades, the famous Greek physician, recommended regular use of chamomile, while in Rome it was used as a bitter tonic and blood purifier.

❁ Chamomile tea is a traditional remedy for menstrual cramp. In France it was drunk for digestion after a meal, and to relieve pain. It is often recommended by modern herbalists for women's nervous conditions, for nervous stomach complaints, and even for dissolving gall stones.

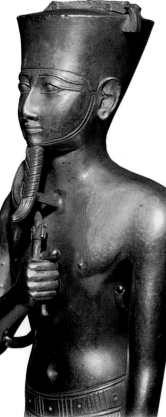

❁ The other major medicinal variety in this family is German chamomile, *Matricaria Chamomilla* or scented mayweed. The major difference is that *Anthemis nobilis* is for nervous disorders, as suggested by its more finely branching leaves. It has smaller flowers and finer toothed leaves that come from the base of the stem rather than branching out.

❁ It it said to be the "plant's physician" because it will revive a drooping plant if put next to it.

LEFT *The Ancient
Egyptians valued
chamomile above all other
herbs and dedicated it to
the sun god Ra.*

CASE STUDY

Melanie, a 40-year-old actress, suffered from bulimia nervosa.
She was quite successful in her career but was getting more bulimic as time went on and finding it difficult to sleep. She felt upset about small things, and she became particularly tense before a performance. She began using Chamomile six times a day.

After she began taking Chamomile, Melanie fell asleep right away; gradually she was able to relax during the day as well. She found that her performances went well and over a six-month period Melanie was able to let go of her anxieties and began to eat normally again.

Anthopleura elegantissima

Sea Anemone

THE SEA *anemone is a marine animal that belongs to the family of* Cnidaria, *which all have stinging cells and move by using their muscles. Shapeless blobs out of water, they are like beautiful flowers under it – sea flowers. Bach included rock water as one of his 38 remedies to help soften those who are too hard on themselves. Sea anemone is included in this flower essence pharmacy because it also works with this type of person, but it is especially important because of its usefulness in dealing directly and immediately with physical pain.*

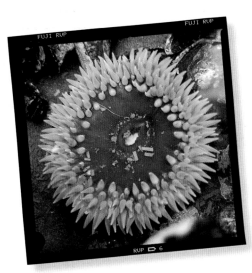

ABOVE *The sea anemone has stinging tentacles that poison its prey.*

❧ *Reduces pain through openness and surrender* ❧

Name
Antho means a flower in Greek, and *anthopleura* means the "flowering of the linings of the lungs." *Elegantissima* is graceful refinement and elegance.

If it were possible to turn our lungs inside out, they would look like flowers, and the pleural membranes would be the petals. The name of sea anemone suggests that it is opening to the world in vulnerable beauty, like lungs turning inside out.

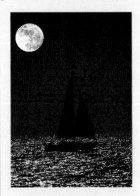

ABOVE *As a creature of the sea, the anemone is believed to be in complete tune with nature's cycles.*

Color/shape
The center of a sea anemone is pink with green outside – colors that nourish the heart. Overall it looks like an eye with large lashes, and it does help us see what is going on.

Habitat and growth pattern
The anemone has a tubelike body attached by the base to a rock or shell.

Its stinging tentacles capture crustaceans and other small organisms – so it has a strong connection to pain.

The anemone's action in the ocean is like breathing in and out. It sways from side to side in sensitive response to the movement of the water. Yet when it is approached it curls in upon itself in an act of self-protection, losing its vulnerability and openness.

FOLKLORE AND USAGE

❀ The tides of the ocean are governed by the phases of the moon, so sea creatures are seen as being in complete harmony with natural cycles. The sea itself represents the cosmic ocean from which we all emerged and to which we will all return. Our body consists of 80 percent water and is also influenced by the moon's phases. So sea anemone helps us give way to profound processes that are much greater than we are and, as such, usually beyond our consciousness.

CASE STUDY

Marcia, a 25-year-old journalist, suffered from insomnia, eye strain, pains in the neck and arms, and tension in her solar plexus.
She felt very angry and thought that her body had really let her down. It was clear to anyone else, however, that it was she who was dominating and controlling her body to meet her ambitious goals. She worked hard in the office and often took work home, which meant that she was frequently awake in the middle of the night, becoming out of tune with her natural cycle.

After one week of taking Sea Anemone, Marcia began to have flashbacks to when she was a child. Her mother told her that she was a "lazy good-for-nothing," who was "lucky to be born." Marcia had always worked as hard as possible just to prove her mother wrong. But until she took sea anemone essence, Marcia had been completely unaware of this.

After another two weeks of Sea Anemone essence, Marcia found she wanted to go to sleep more and felt unaccountably relaxed and carefree. She described feeling as though she were being moved by the ocean, surrendering to and opening up to deeper breathing. But these feelings also frightened her a good deal.

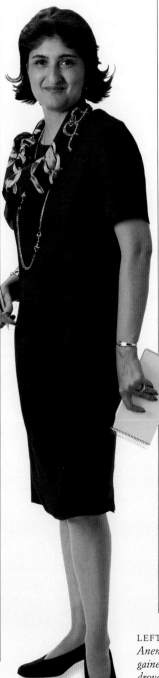

She then developed what seemed like a bad cold. As she struggled with it, she realized that she felt she had to justify almost every breath she took and was never able just to be, but now she couldn't do anything else but lie in bed and rest. This made her feel very vulnerable, not being able "to get on with things" but she heard a voice inside her saying, "love yourself, it'll be all right." Gradually she succumbed to it, telling herself she was convalescing from a lifetime's stress.

But to Marcia's surprise, even when she was better she still took time off to pamper herself with an aromatherapy massage. She felt that her "body was in control now" and seemed like a "new voice" inside her telling her what it wanted – very different from the past when she told it what to do for her.

Continuing with Sea Anemone, after another month she was sleeping well, feeling good, working a normal 40-hour week, and the pains that she had been experiencing in her neck and shoulders had disappeared.

LEFT *After taking Sea Anemone, Marcia felt that she gained an insight into what drove her, opening her heart to a gentler way of being.*

AFFIRMATION
I respond with trust and openness to each moment.

Key words
POSITIVE: *Surrender, empowerment.*
NEGATIVE: *Overachieving, competitiveness, pain, muscle spasm.*

Challenge
To let go of ego control on your life so that your body can attune to deep cycles for healing.

NOTES

Therapeutic actions
It is very useful for physical pain; allows the freedom to move into the pain, instead of resisting it (this in itself reduces the pain's intensity); helps with eye problems and seeing ourselves and our lives with responsibility.

Method of making essence
Sun method.

Ways of using and use in combination
Best used alone; use in an ointment massaged onto strained body parts.

Best supportive technique
Take time off just to be.

Banksia menziesii

Menzies Banksia

THERE ARE *70 or so species of* banksia *that belong to* Proteaceae. *This is one of the most prominent plant families in the southern hemisphere, and it includes the* Proteas *and* Grevilleas *families. It grows in South America, South Africa, and Australia. Many of the species live in near-drought conditions but a few ancestral species live in rain forests. The* banksias *are evergreen trees and shrubs that like temperate to tropical scrub and forest, mainly in Australia. They are cultivated for their attractive foliage and flowers. Many of them are yellow, but this one is red.* Menzies banksia *is also the most untidy – the leaves being toothed in an irregular pattern. It sacrifices formality for vibrancy.*

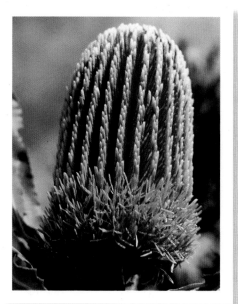

LEFT *The flowerhead of the Menzies banksia contains approximately 1,000 individual reddish flowers.*

❧ *Triumph over disaster leads to renewed energy* ❧

Name
It is also known as firewood banksia. *Banksia* **is named after the botanist Joseph Banks.** *Menziesii* **comes from Menzies, a local collector in the early days of Australia's history.**

Color/shape
Each conelike flower head comprises 1,000 individual flowers. The cones are brushlike; on the subtle level they clear away the debris of painful past experience.
   Menzies banksia **is insignificant in stature compared to other** *banksias***, and is often unsightly in appearance. It blooms in the fall when the reddish flowers begin to open from the base. Gradually taking their time, sometimes taking weeks, row after row of flowers open until the flowering reaches the top of the cone, looking like splendid candles on a Christmas tree. Given time, we can all grow into our potential no matter what sufferings we have had to endure.**

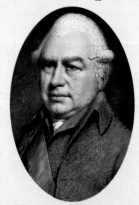

ABOVE *The* Menzies banksia *species is named for the English naturalist Sir Joseph Banks (1743–1820).*

Habitat and growth pattern
Bushfires can be extremely dangerous in Australia, often dimming the sun as far as 1,000 miles away in New Zealand. These trees need to be able to live with fire. In fact the tough wooden seed pods stay tightly shut until the heat of a bushfire bursts them open, throwing the seeds into the newly laid ash to await the first rains. Therefore, the *Menzies banksia* **species thrives on past misfortune.**

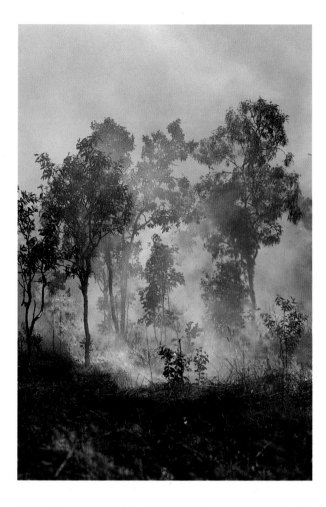

AFFIRMATION
I am free from past hurt and ready to meet my future.

Key words
POSITIVE: *Courage to release pain and to move ahead triumphantly.*
NEGATIVE: *Painful disappointment, deeply held body tension, fear of repeating experience.*

Challenge
To release tension that keeps body and mind from moving freely forward.

LEFT *The seed pods of the* Menzies banksia *trees stay closed until the heat of a bushfire forces them open.*

Cynthia, a 40-year-old, had had a very painful end to a relationship. She fell ill with chronic fatigue syndrome. Her muscles hurt and she felt so bad about herself that she wanted to retreat from the world entirely. She lost trust in most of the other people around her and was unable to confide in anyone, even in her closest friends. She felt trapped in her pain and believed that any affection she was given might be withdrawn at any time.

After some time of using *Menzies banksia* essence Cynthia was able to tackle her disappointment and began to be able to tell her friends about her painful experience in love and discuss what was happening to her body. Gradually she started to be able to do a little exercise, which helped release some of the stress from her muscles. Local application of the essence helped ease the muscle pain. With the help of acupuncture and counseling, she gradually recovered from her emotional blow and developed a new relationship. She is currently making good progress in recovering from chronic fatigue syndrome.

NOTES

Therapeutic actions
Helps us to let go of past hurt in relationships and to find a new future with faith; on the physical level, temporarily helps soothe intense localized pain in muscle and soft tissue; helps to keep the body relaxed when you anticipate future pain because of past experience; for back pain, it can be rubbed over the outer ear with a Q-tip that has been dipped in the stock essence.

Method of making essence
Sun method.

Ways of using and use in combination
Take from dosage bottle night and morning; for the body, apply stock dilution directly to the painful area; use in the bath to relieve muscle pain.

Best supportive technique
Bodywork to discover what is being held in the muscles; polarity therapy; reiki; biodynamics.

BELOW *Use Menzies Banksia essence on a Q-tip and rub over the affected area to relieve back pain.*

Borago officinalis

Borage

BORAGE *belongs to the forget-me-not* (Boraginacea) *family that grows mostly in rocky places in western, central, and eastern Europe, and the Mediterranean. Borago officinalis came originally from Italy but is now naturalized in most parts of Europe. It has long been grown as a medicinal herb and because it is an excellent source of nectar for bees.*

LEFT *Borage will attract honey bees to your garden.*

ABOVE *The attractive flowers of the borage plant consist of five blue petals surrounding a hub of black stamens.*

SIGNATURE

❧ *Keep moving with courage* ❧

Name
Borage is a corruption of the Latin *corago* from *cor*, the heart, and *ago*, I bring, because of its cordial effect as an herb. It could also be derived from *barrach*, a Celtic word which means "a man of courage."

Color/shape
Borage's five-petaled flower, 1in. (2.5cm) across, is a translucent brilliant cobalt blue color, sometimes tinged with magenta. The sepals form another green five-pointed star behind it. The delicate blue color of the flower contrasts with all the other parts of the plant, which are rough and hairy. The borage flower is shaped like a wheel, with the black anthers forming a hub in the center.

BORAGO OFFICINALIS

Habitat and growth pattern
Borage is a really robust plant that grows well in dry places. It will do well even in a cold summer. It seeds freely and can grow to 18in. (45cm) across.

ABOVE *Originally from Italy, borage is now found all over Europe and the Mediterranean.*

AFFIRMATION

I have the courage and strength to enjoy my life and move forward, whatever may come.

Key words

POSITIVE: *Buoyant courage and optimism.*
NEGATIVE: *Down-hearted, broken-hearted, pessimism.*

Challenge

To find strength and courage whatever the circumstances.

CASE STUDY

Jim was setting up a new business but he had not realized just how much effort it would take.

He was used to working in a team and sharing the problems that arose every day, so he soon grew very disheartened and eventually became ill with bronchitis. This persisted for three months. He was on the verge of giving up his new business but really didn't know what else to do. He was given massage and plenty of Borage. Within two weeks he was back at work with much greater optimism about its eventual success.

NOTES

Therapeutic actions
Alleviates discouragement; brings cheerfulness to face the trials of life; useful in cases of long-term sickness and other trying or difficult circumstances.

Method of making essence
Sun method.

Ways of using and use in combination
Dosage bottle, in baths; useful with any other flower essence.

Best supportive technique
Share your troubles with a friend; deep aerobic breathing, with or without strenuous exercise; keep in good physical condition and use the healing properties of the physical plant too. If you have a borage plant, pick the leaves and cook them, and use the flowers to liven up a salad. If not, buy the oil.

BELOW *Borage herb acts on the endocrine system, so it is a good remedy to take for hormonal problems.*

ABOVE RIGHT *The Roman scientist Pliny (23–79 C.E.) wrote in his* Natural History *that borage gave courage.*

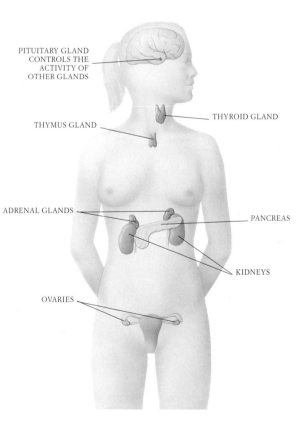

PITUITARY GLAND CONTROLS THE ACTIVITY OF OTHER GLANDS

THYMUS GLAND

THYROID GLAND

ADRENAL GLANDS

PANCREAS

KIDNEYS

OVARIES

FOLKLORE AND USAGE

❁ Pliny said that borage brought courage, while in the late 17th century John Evelyn said, "Sprigs of Borage are of known virtue to revive the hypochondriac and cheer the hard student." The blue flowers used to be candied "for the comfort of the heart and to drive away sorrow."

❁ Borage acts on the adrenal glands and does increase courage.

❁ Borage contains similar oils to evening primrose. These feed the hormonal system, which has a very important influence on our moods. It is sold as starflower oil.

❁ Young fresh borage leaves have a high concentration of vitamin C, and leaves chopped up in salad strengthen the nervous system. They smell and taste like fresh cucumbers and can be used as "herbal ice" to cool summer drinks.

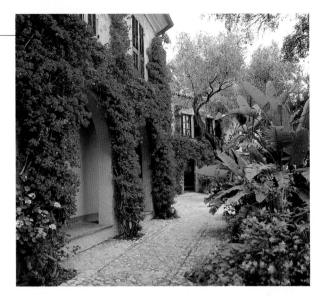

Bougainvillea spectabilis

Bougainvillea

T HE BOUGAINVILLEA *or* Nytaginaceae *family is made up chiefly of herbs, shrubs, and trees found throughout the tropics, particularly in America. It also contains* Mirabilis *and* Pisonia, *which are cultivated as vegetables.* Bougainvillea spectabilis *is a South American tropical vine now naturalized in warm countries throughout the world for the vivid red and purple bracts that cover the flowers. In the United States it grows over the walls of New Orleans homes. This particular bougainvillea blooms in January, when the light is beginning to return.*

ABOVE RIGHT *The climbing bougainvillea plant adds a glorious splash of color to many homes.*

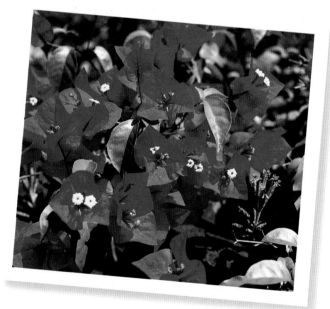

ABOVE *Bougainvillea is a spectacular climbing shrub that can be found throughout the tropics.*

SIGNATURE

❦ *Unconditional love shatters the illusion of guilt* ❧

Name
Bougainville was an 18th-century French navigator. The Latin *spectabilis* means spectacular.

Color/shape
The inconspicuous, tubular flowers shine like three little white stars enfolded in a vivid cloak of color. All bougainvillea's fertile parts are inside the three unified tubular petals. So it is deeply self-contained in modest white. This inward quality contrasts with the most colorful parts of the bougainvillea – the three flamboyant magenta bracts that shelter the flowers. The number three has long been a "holy" number, representing the union of body, mind, and spirit, or the Christian Trinity – the Father, Son, and Holy Ghost. This vivid magenta is the color that emanates from the spiritual center above the top of our heads, so it is deeply nourishing to the spirit. So spiritual nourishment that comes from above unifies, protects, and enlivens humility. Humility is very different from guilt, but we can confuse the issue when we are depressed.

Habitat and growth pattern
Bougainvillea is a hardy vine, often thorny, that grows in tropical climates and climbs with spectacular abundance. It makes festoons of color throughout forests, over walls, and over other trees and shrubs.

During the day the bracts shine, but at night the flowers attract moths. In Eastern culture the moth is a symbol of sacrificial love, because it is drawn to the light, willing to die in the purifying flames.

Key words

POSITIVE: *Awareness of spiritual love and protection, self-forgiveness.*
NEGATIVE: *Living in fear, perfectionism, guilt.*

Challenge

To enjoy the abundance of love revealed in creation.

AFFIRMATION
I am filled with the magic and splendor of life.

CASE STUDY

Jeremy had painful knotted shoulders and neck. Nothing, including massage or osteopathy, seemed to bring him much relief.

He had deep furrows between his eyebrows and a constant pain behind his eyes. After taking Bougainvillea he gradually felt able to tell his story.

Jeremy lived in fear of being punished for every wrong thought or mistake he had ever made; he felt so guilty that he could never enjoy his successes.

He awarded himself points for good behavior but they were simply offset against the bad points he had awarded himself. Two months after beginning to take Bougainvillea, Jeremy began to experience life quite differently. He appreciated that he did a good job and worked hard.

Now he felt able to enjoy the encouragement offered by his wife. His garden became a source of pleasure and he no longer felt the necessity to work in it all the time. Walks in the country lifted his spirits still further, and the furrows in his forehead went away.

HIS MENTAL MOOD LIGHTENED

THE PAIN IN HIS SHOULDERS AND NECK EASED

THE DEEP FURROWS IN HIS FOREHEAD DISAPPEARED

JEREMY BEGAN TO WALK FREELY

LEFT *After taking Bougainvillea flower essence for a few months, Jeremy felt his spirits lighten and he began to enjoy refreshing walks.*

NOTES

Therapeutic actions
Realigns emotions to the spirit and releases guilt and fear of reprisal by connecting with the force of love; makes us appreciative of life's pleasures; makes us willing to aid others to feel comfortable and welcome, even in the most difficult situations; deepens breathing and encourages feelings of peace and ease; reduces local aches and pains, including chronic pain; good for chronic fatigue.

Method of making essence
Sun method.

Ways of using and use in combination
Combines well with Impatiens or Dandelion for pain and spasms. Make into a lotion and apply all over the body, following the meridian system, especially lung and colon points; apply locally, two drops may be put directly onto unbroken skin.

Best supportive technique
Establish habits that are rewarding and pleasurable, including regular meditation.

Bromus ramosus

Wild Oat

WILD OAT *is a member of the grass family* (Graminacea), *which is distributed throughout the world. There are more than 8,000 known species. Grains like wheat, oats, rye, barley, and millet are major staple foods around the world. Durable grasses hold the earth together, keeping it free from erosion, and are also used for cultivated lawns. So clearly the grasses are of the greatest service to humankind. Wild oat is native to most of Europe, North Africa, North America, and temperate Asia. It is found in hedgerows, woods, and shady places throughout Britain. It is sometimes sown in pastures as forage.*

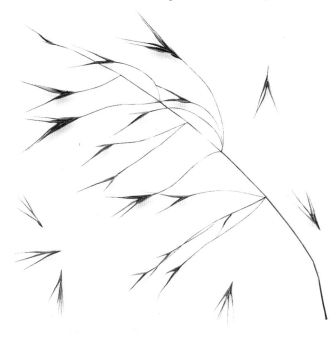

ABOVE *Although of nutritional value, the wild oat is not commonly harvested as a food source.*

SIGNATURE

❧ *Willingness to serve makes the path clearer* ❧

Name
Wild oat is also called hairy brome or wood brome. *Bromus* **is a latinization of the classical Greek word for oat.** *Ramosus* **means branching, so it is a branching oat.**

Color/shape
Wild oat is a perennial, with a tall stem that can grow to over 4ft. (1.25m). Because they have wind-pollinated flowers, grasses do not need bright petals to attract insects. So the stiff open flowerheads have such small dull green flowers that you may not even see them.

The energy required for a showy flower is used instead to increase its food value.

Habitat and growth pattern
The loose panicle of flowers hangs down, flopping and waving around in every direction as the wind blows. Members of the grass family are naturally useful plants to humankind, providing food and helping to prevent soil erosion, but the wild oat has not yet found its role in this type of service, being scattered and not easily harvested.

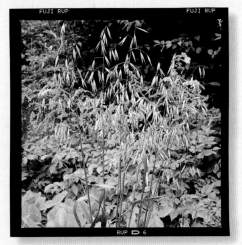

ABOVE *A member of the grass family, the wild oat species can grow up to 4ft. (1.25m) high.*

FOLKLORE AND USAGE

❁ "Sowing your wild oats" means to plant your seed in many different locations. The saying is usually applied to young men before they settle down and get married.

Key words

POSITIVE: *Clarity of purpose, contentment.*
NEGATIVE: *Confusion about life direction, chronic dissatisfaction.*

Challenge

To become determined to use your time usefully and satisfyingly.

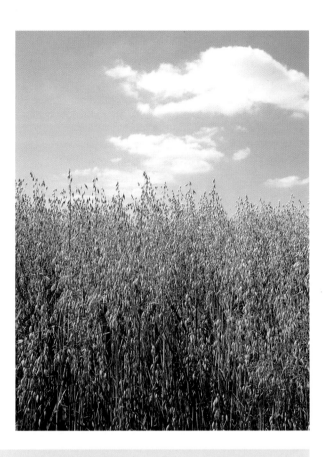

RIGHT *Native to Europe, North Africa, North America, and parts of Asia, wild oat grows in hedgerows.*

CASE STUDY

Jonathan was a 40-year-old intelligent, but restless man. He had many different jobs during his lifetime, none of which fulfiled his potential.
His capabilities were very clear from the deep and varied interests that he had in the health field and the excellent advice he was able to give to friends about their health problems.

During the last few years he'd taken on a steady job as a taxi driver in order to support himself while he trained as a homeopath.

He completed his training successfully, but then found it difficult to get clients. True to type, he began thinking that he should train in another health field in order to increase his skills.

Jonathan was given Wild Oat and he very quickly decided that he shouldn't train any further, but that he needed to put more effort into creating opportunities for business. He decided to rent a room at a new local health clinic, even though there was no business in view at that time. Within two weeks he had seven clients and a year later was successful, settled, and personally satisfied.

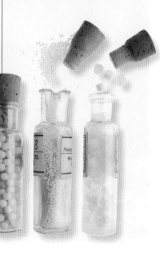

RIGHT *With the help of Wild Oat, Jonathan created a successful homeopathic practice.*

Calliandra eriophylla

Fairy Duster

FAIRY DUSTER *comes from a family often named as powder puff trees. They are the mimosa branch of the pea family,* Leguminosae/ Mimosaceae. *This family is able to fix nitrogen in the soil and thus regenerate it. It includes legumes such as peas and beans, as well as the beautiful brooms. They enjoy a great variety of habitats and include water-loving plants and climbers. This delicate fairy duster blooms in the harshness of lower desert from southern California to southwest and northwest New Mexico and grows in sandy washes and open slopes in deserts and arid grasslands.*

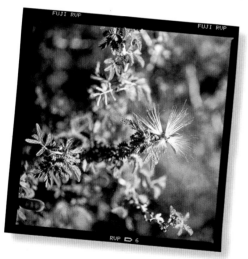

ABOVE *The fairy duster, or angel head, has beautiful and densely packed pinkish-red flowers, with long, feathery stamens.*

SIGNATURE

❦ *Bombardment of the senses is calmed and centered* ❧

Name
Fairy duster is also called angel head. *Calliendrum* **was a headdress worn by Roman women and was built up with false hair;** *eriophorous* **means having a thick cottony covering of hairs. So the Latin name of the plant describes the plant's beautiful stamen and its woolly leaves.**

Color/shape
The flowers are nearly 2in. (5cm) wide and are densely packed. The pinkish-red petals are tiny, with exquisite pink puffs of long stamens that form feathery balls. Between 10 and 100 stamens form a wonderful mandala (a circle enclosing geometric designs), with a center of white exquisitely turning to pink toward the perimeter. The stamens dance responsively to every waft of breeze.

Red is a color of vitality, and white of clarity and purity. The common name of angel head suggests that among all the activity (red) that could unbalance us, soothing white can calm and center us like an angelic force.

Habitat and growth pattern
Desert plants need to conserve energy because they have to deal with a huge variety of stimuli, from extreme drought to torrential rain, and a wide range of temperatures between day and night. The fairy duster conserves its energy during these extremes. But this small contorted shrub, inconspicuous for most of the year, bursts forth as soon as the least moisture is available making its presence known seemingly from out of nowhere.

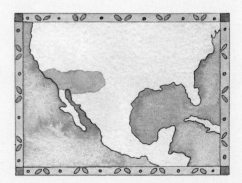

ABOVE *Fairy duster is native to the deserts of California, Arizona and New Mexico.*

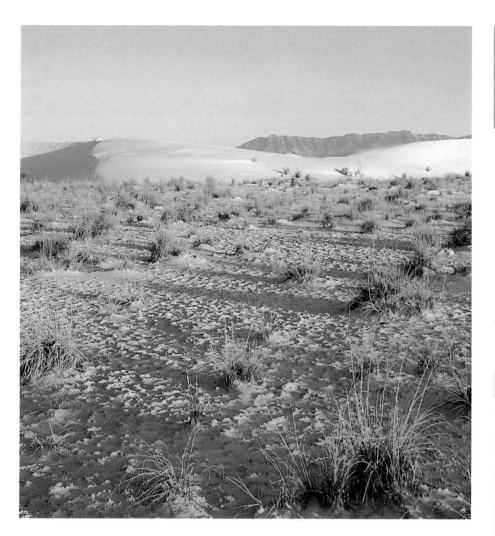

ABOVE *The fairy duster thrives in harsh desert conditions, bursting into flower as soon as moisture becomes available.*

Key words
POSITIVE: *Stability, integration of learning processes, peace.*
NEGATIVE: *Overexcitability, hypersensitivity, nervous system imbalance.*

Challenge
To keep balanced and focused in the center of over-abundant mental stimuli.

CASE STUDY

Nadine worked at home and was feeling under pressure from her work, her family, and her friends. She felt overwhelmed and overstimulated and "didn't have time to catch breath." She took three drops from a stock bottle of Fairy Duster twice daily for two days. By the end of the second day, she had stopped her frantic work pattern and took time to reorganize her environment. A week later she felt that Fairy Duster had helped her to calm down enough to consider her options more creatively. She now had more privacy and a space outdoors to escape to. She was breathing freely again.

NOTES

Therapeutic actions
Fairy Duster soothes those who are overwhelmed by mental stimuli; it helps digest experiences when there is too much to take in; it balances hyperactivity and underactivity; helps to maintain awareness; is effective in many nervous system disorders.

Method of making essence
Sun method.

Ways of using and use in combination
Take three to five drops, as needed; add to bath water; add a few drops to a vaporizer bottle of water and spray into the room; place a few drops directly on the body, especially on any of the chakra areas.

Best supportive technique
While taking the essence, take seven deep and slow inhalations. Giving attention to your breathing is also useful to reduce stress at any time.

Casuarina glauca

She Oak

THE CASUARINACEAE *is a distinctive family of trees and shrubs adapted to the dry habitats of Australia, Malaysia, New Caledonia, Fiji, and the Mascarene Islands. There are approximately 65 species, mostly tall trees very similar to conifers. For this reason, the family is also called river oak, or Australian pine. They are able to conserve moisture remarkably well because of the extreme smallness of their leaves and the deeply grooved and jointed branches. Many members of this family are useful, as lumber for furniture manufacture, for instance, but* Casuarina glauca *is useful to the body's hormone system.*

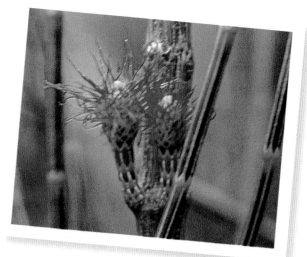

ABOVE *The she oak is a bisexual species that contains both male and female flowers on different parts of the plant.*

SIGNATURE

❦ *Confidence in the enduring ability to create life* ❧

Name

The name *Casuarina* is from the flightless cassowary bird, whose feathers resemble the drooping branches of the she oak; *glauca* means covered with a "bloom," the fine white powdery coating that a plum has. But this tree's common name, she oak, gives us the greatest clue to its use. It is as strong as the oak but is particularly for use by women.

Color/shape

The female flowers grow in globular heads on which each short style divides into two long lobed stigmas. The stigmas hang out of the flowers to catch pollen on the wind in a very similar way to that in which the fallopian tubes wait to catch the eggs ejected from the ovaries. The male flowers are tiny and petalless and are borne in densely packed conelike spikes at the ends of the plant's branches.

The seeds have an embryo and no endosperm, because they are strong enough to survive without a protective covering.

Habitat and growth pattern

Although it lives by streams and wetlands, the she oak is supremely adapted to coping with the inevitable droughts in very dry regions of high temperature and low rainfall. The stem photosynthesizes rather than the leaves, which are extremely small, like minute scales or teeth arranged in a collarlike ring at each node to save evaporation. *Casuarina* is bisexual with male and female flowers growing on different parts of the plant, and it relies on the wind for pollination.

FOLKLORE AND USAGE

✿ Biologists used to think that casuarinas were distinct and independent from all other flowering plant families, and that they were extremely primitive, but now they are inclined to think that the peculiar features of this family are the result of extreme specializations in isolated conditions. Whichever is true, this plant knows how to continue the species and procreate!

CASE STUDY

Margaret came to flower essence therapy because she was feeling tired and run down. She was going through her menopause and often felt aggressive and short-tempered. Her husband had not approached her to make love for some time, which made her very distressed. When they had made love during the early part of her menopause it had been physically difficult and this had put them both off. She felt unsure about approaching her husband sexually since he was often tired from working long hours.

After taking She Oak for a couple of weeks, Margaret began to have romantic dreams, her temper calmed, her skin felt softer, and she felt generally sweeter. She found herself dressing in more feminine clothes, which attracted her husband. She realized that having had three unplanned pregnancies made her worry about having another one. She knew it was now impossible for her conceive and began to relax more. Her husband also began to take the essence. After another month they returned to a happy sex life.

NOTES

Therapeutic actions
Overcomes hormonal imbalances in females, therefore is a useful alternative to HRT if taken with appropriate professional advice; balances testosterone in men; helps in coping with distress associated with infertility and difficult sex.

Method of making essence
Sun method, possibly combined with boiling method.

Ways of using and use in combination
For infertility, take seven drops in a dosage bottle night and morning for four weeks, leave two weeks then repeat the cycle four more times. If conception has not occurred after six months then add Flannel Flower (see p. 139 for suppliers).

Best supportive technique
Look at any childhood difficulties that may have caused a deep distress about birth, such as your mother or father not wanting your conception.

(see p. 139 for suppliers)

Key words
POSITIVE: *Reproduction, conception.*
NEGATIVE: *Hormonal imbalance in females, unable to conceive, difficult sex.*

Challenge
To face and overcome blocks, whether conscious or unconscious that prevent conception.

AFFIRMATION
I create new life confidently.

MAY BE USED INSTEAD OF HRT (WITH APPROPRIATE PROFESSIONAL ADVICE)

REDUCES STRESS ASSOCIATED WITH INFERTILITY

AIDS CONCEPTION

HELPS BALANCE TESTOSTERONE

RIGHT *She Oak is a good remedy for hormonal imbalance, particularly concerning infertility.*

Cichorium intybus

Chicory

CHICORY *is a member of the* Asteracea *branch of the sunflower family. It is native to Europe, western Asia, and North Africa. It has been introduced to much of the world including North America. It is widespread and common throughout the British Isles, except in the far north. It grows on roadsides, waste places, and dry banks. This chicory should not be confused with the endive* Chicorium endivia, *which is cultivated for salads.*

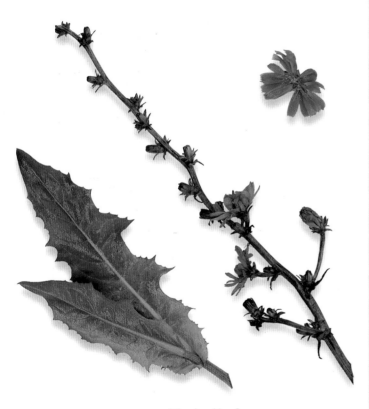

ABOVE *The clear blue flowers of the chicory plant are very distinctive and grow on stems up to 5ft. (1.5m) high.*

SIGNATURE

🌿 *Abundant universal love creates detached caring* 🌺

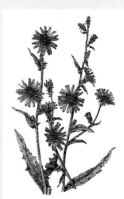

CICHORIUM INTYBUS

Name
It is also known as blue succory, monk's beard, hard ewes, or strip for strip. It is called succory from the Latin *succurere*, to run under, because of the depth to which the root penetrates.

Color/shape
Chicory is a tall perennial with vivid sky-blue flowers that are up to 1.5in. (4cm) in diameter. The chicory blue is very striking and indicates its healing qualities clearly. Just as blue is the color of the sky and the ocean, which are the vast spaces of the planet and the universe, so chicory is concerned with the generosity of giving space to others. Not only that, it also betokens spiritual love, a calming love that sees everything and forgives all. Choosing blue above other colors indicates a desire for order and peace.

The flowers are held close to the stem, like stars that have been pinned on. Although the petals are ragged, the pale indigo styles are erect. Chicory suggests fragility mixed with strength, with its fragile ragged-looking petals contrasting with the strong indigo styles pointing straight up. The flowers also have two sets of bracts for protection. The flowers wilt quickly when you pick them but they are truly prolific. Chicory can flower for four months, with around 2,000 blooms in its lifetime, and can grow to 5ft. (1.5m).

Habitat and growth pattern
The tap root system is enormous, at least as large as the flowering plant. This underground strength anchors it and allows the generous giving of its flowers.

Chicory has tough hairy grooved stems and leaves that form a rosette at the base of the plant. The lobed and toothed leaves grip the stem tightly, just as we hold on tightly to those we love.

Key words

POSITIVE: *Generous love, emotional clarity, respect of others' need for freedom.*
NEGATIVE: *Emotional fragility, neediness, possessiveness, insecurity, manipulation.*

Challenge

To know the source of universal love within yourself; to love others unconditionally.

CASE STUDY

Caroline, a 50-year-old, fell downstairs and hurt her spine badly.
After taking Chicory she realized that the accident was an unconscious attempt to gain attention from her 20-year-old son because she was upset by his growing independence. Gradually Caroline became less dependent and her son felt free and able to leave home. He could now develop a good relationship with his mother.

FOLKLORE AND USAGE

❊ There are many legends about chicory. In Germany there is a story that a young girl mourning the death of her lover continued to weep until she sank into the ground whereupon chicory grew up from the spot. Another legend says that the flowers are the tears of a woman with beautiful blue eyes whose lover never returned. Consequently it was traditionally used in love potions or to help forget a lost love.

❊ Chicory flowers open and close at set times each day, around 7:00 a.m. to 12:00 noon. According to another legend, a gentle lady named Florilor was transformed into a chicory plant when she rejected the advances of the sun god. To this day, in her altered form she mocks him, turns her face to him until noon, then closes her flowers and ignores him.

❊ Chicory has been used as a blood purifier, a laxative, tonic, and for animals and humans for jaundice and liver complaints. It was recommended to prevent paralyzed limbs from wasting. Used in salad, the bitter taste of the leaves tones up the digestive system. When used as a medicinal herb it strengthens the physical body. As a flower essence it gives independence and greater strength to our emotions.

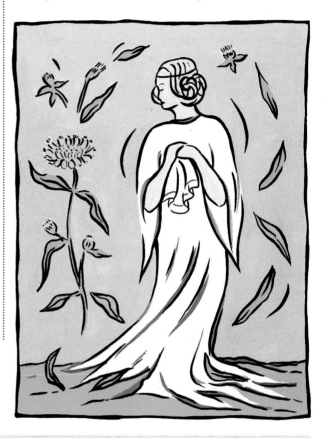

RIGHT *Many legends concerning chicory relate to lost love.*

NOTES

Therapeutic actions
Gives an experience of self-contained emotional nourishment; helps to overcome feelings of neediness and emptiness, therefore, is very useful in eating disorders; excellent for adults and children who are needy, over-demanding, or behave manipulatively.

Method of making essence
Sun method. Use only the wild plant. Pick flowers that are intensely blue. They fade quickly so you may only have enough time to pick two or three flowerheads.

Ways of using and use in combination
Good with Bleeding Heart.

Best supportive technique
Befriending the inner child, so that you can understand and know more directly what it is that you need rather than using unconscious manipulation.

Clematis vitalba

Clematis

CLEMATIS VITALBA *belongs to the Crowfoot or* Ranunculacea *family, which is a wideranging group, of great botanical interest. It is a large family containing well-known wild flowers such as buttercups, anemones, and hellebores. There are 300 species of clematis worldwide growing in Europe, the Himalayas, China, Australia, North and Central America. They differ widely. There are short-growing herbaceous perennials, trailing shrubs, and climbers that reach 50ft. (15m) high. The great color range of their large sepals and a long flowering period make them attractive and popular garden plants.*

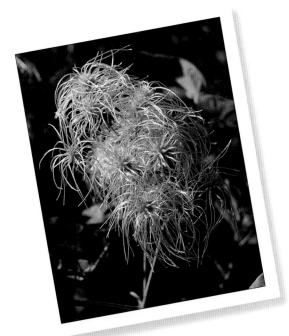

ABOVE *The clematis belongs to the same family as some well-known wild flowers, such as buttercups and hellebores.*

SIGNATURE

🌼 *Cling fast to the present so that you can realize your dreams* 🌼

Name
Clematis means a vine-shoot because the stem twists and turns like the vine. *Vitalba* means full of white from *alba* (white) and *vita* (life). It was called Travelers Joy by John Gerard because it grows profusely in hedgerows along the roadside. The downy seeds wing their way through the air. Another nickname – old man's beard – refers to the downy heads of the fruit.

Color/shape
The greenish-white flowers grow in large groups on the ends of branchlets. There are no petals but four to six thick white tongue-shaped sepals, which are furry, and a number of creamy stamens. Their pale green styles grow into long silvery threadlike tails that form the distinctive white hairy masses.

Habitat and growth pattern
Clematis is a straggling climber that drapes itself over hedges, in clouds of white plumed fruits and gives an amorphous looking silvery-gray cloudy appearance. Head in the clouds, they seem to have no focus of attention, no direction. But in fact, Clematis twines itself around other plants with a vicelike grip clinging on right through the fall. This shows its real power to hold on as and when necessary.

As it grows old its many stems can twist together, forming a strong cable – a real strength to deal with life. Interestingly it grows on chalky soil, calcium being very essential for alert brain functioning. Also the clematis fragrance is of almonds, which are excellent brain food.

FOLKLORE AND USAGE

❋ Also called the baccy plant, smokewood, or woodbine because the dry winter stems have been cut for smoking.

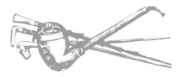

ABOVE *The dried stems of the clematis plant were added to pipe tobacco for smoking.*

Key words

POSITIVE: *Alert to the present, realizing vision.*
NEGATIVE: *Daydreaming, ungrounded, impractical.*

Challenge

To convert your dreams and visions into practical reality.

ABOVE *One of the most relaxing and pleasant ways of using Clematis is to add it to your bath essence.*

NOTES

Therapeutic actions
Enables the conversion of dreams into practical action. Draws all aspects of a person into the present including thoughts, feelings, and emotions so that more satisfying contact with others is possible. Helps to deal with escapism that leads to over-frequent drug taking. Clematis helps avert physical illness caused by not being fully present in the body.

Method of making essence.
Sun method.

Ways of using and use in combination
Use in dosage bottle, in ointments, in baths.

Best supportive technique
Walking or running, to bring energy and awareness into the body. Breathing or other awareness practice. Determine to complete unfinished business.

CASE STUDY

Wendy had a history of frequent tonsillitis. She was an idealist – always full of plans for improving her life.
She was always "going to" do a million things: to go on a diet; to decorate to lift up her spirits; to organize the kitchen. But somehow things remained the same – she stayed overweight and always in a muddle.

After taking clematis for two weeks she stopped spending time thinking about ways to change her life and began to take action. She sorted out the garage and found lots of paints she could start decorating with right away. Instead of taking drugs for her sore throat she fasted on fruit juices and then amended her diet to raw foods only, a regimen she followed for three months. She used Clematis regularly over a couple of years and began to realize that she could fulfil many more of her dreams, including gardening, which she found both therapeutic and pleasurable. She suffered no further bouts of tonsillitis.

SHE NO LONGER HAD TONSILLITIS

SHE LOST WEIG GRADUALLY

RIGHT *Clematis essence helped to make Wendy's dreams concrete as well as improve her health.*

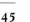

Crowea saligna

Crowea

CROWEA SALIGNA *belongs to the Citrus fruit family or* Rutaceae, *which loves the tropical and warm temperate countries of Africa and Australia. It is one of three species of evergreen shrub and woody perennials found in scrub and open woodland in New South Wales, Australia. The plants in this family are of enormous value for the lemons, oranges, and other citrus foods that they provide. Often, too, the small oil glands on the back of the leaves give us perfumes.* Ruta graveolens *gives this family its name and the homeopathic remedy that is used for sprains and injuries. It is equally beneficial for the peace of mind it can give us.*

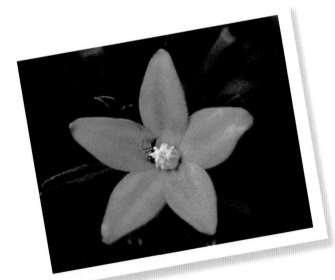

ABOVE *The crowea has pretty star-shaped pink flowers. These flowers are made up of five petals, the number of the senses.*

SIGNATURE

❧ *The unquiet heart finds balance* ❧

Name
It is sometimes called willow-leaved crowea. James Crowe was an 18th-century botanist from Norwich, England, who specialized in collecting willows. *Salignus* **means made of willow-wood.**

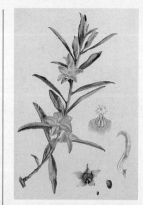

CROWEA SALIGNA

Color/shape
Crowea's magenta pink flowers are star-shaped with five wide-open spreading petals. Five is the number of the senses, and pink the color that nourishes the heart. The flowers are often greenish on the outside – another color that nourishes the heart. Each flower has ten stamens with bearded anthers that add to the vitality of its appearance. The number ten represents completeness and groundedness. These petals have a waxy coating that helps to protect them from the heat of the sun, preventing moisture loss. In the same way, crowea can keep us from losing our cool too.

Habitat and growth pattern
Crowea grows in rocky, sandy sites on the coast and tablelands of central New South Wales. The bush has many open branches of deep green narrow leaves. Each leaf-joint holds a single flower, as if to protect it.

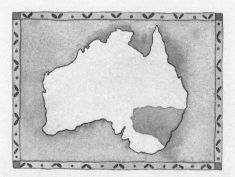

ABOVE *Crowea grows in the open woodland and scrub of New South Wales.*

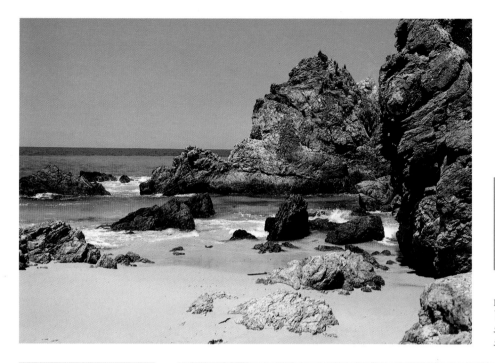

Key words
POSITIVE: *Peace, calm.*
NEGATIVE: *Worry, anxiety.*

Challenge
*Take care of yourself deeply,
so that you have ample
energy and vitality for
present tasks.*

AFFIRMATION
I am serene and fully
aware in all my senses.

LEFT *Native to New South
Wales in Australia, the crowea
shrub thrives in rocky and
sandy conditions.*

CASE STUDY

**Victoria, a middle-aged
woman who was
progressing in her
career, found it very
difficult to cope with
the added level of stress
caused by her increased
contact with the
business world.**
She found she had
endless worries about
whether she was getting
it right. She was also
belching a lot. After
taking Crowea for a few
days, Victoria was able
to find her strength and
tackle issues head on.
She needed fewer treats
to "keep her going"
and consequently her
digestion improved.

NOTES

Therapeutic actions
*All meridians, organs, and
muscles are strengthened
and balanced by crowea;
gives peace and calm, and
therefore, helps with
stomach acidity and all
problems that are to do
with digestion and the
nervous system.*

**Method of
making essence**
Sun method.

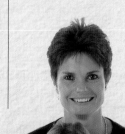

RIGHT *Crowea
flower essence
helps us to give
love generously.*

**Ways of using and
use in combination**
*Seven drops under the tongue
straight from the stock bottle
help align the energy system
to its optimum functioning.*

*Use twice daily, first thing
in the morning and last
thing at night, on a regular
basis. It is used in the Bush
Essences' Emergency,
Travel, Dynamis, and
Radiation formulas.
Refer to Combining and
Combinations (see pp.
124–5). Use Crowea with
Silver Princess to help you
know what it is that you
really want.*

Best supportive technique
*Get to know your inner
child and find out what
might be troubling him or
her. Learn to hold him or
her by the hand; do some
enjoyable aerobic
exercise each day.*

Dampiera linearis

Dampiera

THE Goodeniaceae *family grow mainly as herbs, undershrubs, and occasionally as shrubs. Some of them are deciduous and some evergreen. It is a small family consisting of Brunonia, Scaevola, Goodenia, and Dampiera. They enjoy the heath and high mountain habitats of Australia, growing there almost exclusively. The flowers are usually yellow, blue, or sometimes white. Many popular ornamentals also belong to this family, including Leschnaultia.*

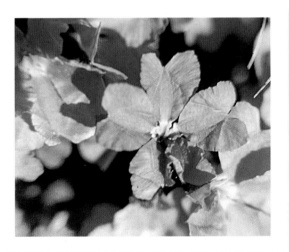

ABOVE *Composed of five petals, the dampiera flower is a cooling blue color.*

Name

Dampier was an English explorer who landed on the west Australian coast in 1688. *Linearis* **means narrow; with its nearly parallel sides, it is almost geometrically perfect.**

Color/shape

Dampiera has five-petaled, blue flowers 0.5in. (1.5cm) across, in cymes that grow to 2in. (5cm) long in the summer. The number five relates to the senses, and blue is a cooling and thoughtful color, so dampiera helps us to release anxious thoughts about what impacts on our senses.

Habitat and growth pattern

Their fruits are nutlike but they don't open even when they are ripe, indicating a reluctance to open up to life. But the plant flowers prolifically in the spring from tiny little cracks in the ground. It shows its real strength by reproducing through suckers as well as seeds. It remains free from pests and diseases, even out of its normal habitat.

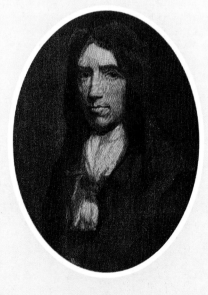

ABOVE *The* dampiera *species is named for William Dampier, the 17th-century English explorer.*

AFFIRMATION
I let go of perfectionism and thoroughly enjoy myself here and now.

Key words
POSITIVE: *Perspective, at ease, relaxed.*
NEGATIVE: *Finicky, tense, overconventional.*

Challenge
To be open to the flow of life, within and without, as it is.

CASE STUDY

Cheryl was unable to make love without everything being perfect – music, lights, no distractions, and her husband saying the "right" things.
She became so finicky that her husband gave up wanting to make love to her because he couldn't get it right enough for her. After taking Dampiera for a couple of months, however, Cheryl was able to make love, and she and her husband began to enjoy a happy and relaxed sex life.

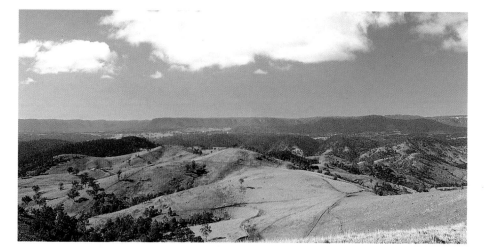

ABOVE *The* Goodeniaceae *family of herbs and shrubs grow in a variety of conditions, from heath to high mountains.*

NOTES

Therapeutic actions
Letting go on any level; helps you to feel less worried by small things and to feel more secure in changing or unfamiliar environments; helps the oversocialized, conventional aspects of yourself to let go and see other points of view; excellent for tight, stressed, or knotted muscles and deep exhaustion.

Method of making essence
Sun method.

Ways of using and use in combination
Dosage bottle; on a Q-tip apply directly onto a tense muscle; use with Dandelion essence.

Best supportive technique
Five rhythms dancing or any free dancing. Remember that life is extremely short.

BELOW *Dampiera essence helps us to relax so that we may let ourselves go and enjoy our relationships.*

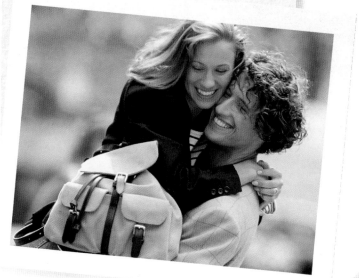

Dicentra formosa

Bleeding Heart

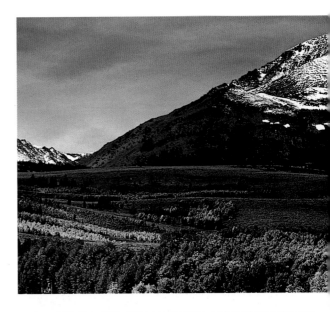

BLEEDING HEART *belongs to the Fumitory family containing 20 or more species of annuals and perennials that grow from Asia to North America. They like the moisture of woodland, and are to be found growing mostly in the mountains. The delicate flowers of* Dicentra formosa *bloom wild around the Sierra Nevada crest in western North America from March until July. There are a few garden varieties that grow well in Europe, though it is the showier* Dicentra spectabilis *that is best known.*

Other wild forms of Dicentra, *like shorthorn steershead and longhorn steershead, do not have the same strong heart shape.*

BELOW *Bleeding heart is so called on account of its flowers that look like a heart that has been cut in two.*

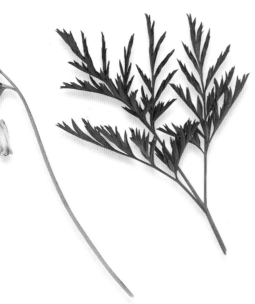

SIGNATURE

❧ *The heart releases its wounds* ❧

Name
Other names include lady in the bath, locket flower, and wild bleeding heart. *Dicentra* suggests two parts around a center, and *formosa* means beautiful and finely formed.

Color/shape
Of all the flowers this must be the clearest in its signature. In the spring the slim stems make graceful arches that dangle rows of small heart-shaped deep rose-pink buds, raised high above the foliage. As they open, the four rose-pink petals in two unlike pairs make a flattened heart shape. If one were to take the two upturned points at the bottom of the heart and bring them together it would make a classical heart shape. As it is, however, the flower looks as though a surgeon has taken a scalpel and slit up from the bottom point of the heart and pushed the wings back to let it bleed – thus bleeding heart.

Habitat and growth pattern
The slender stem, and the much-divided lacy leaves look fragile – as though the heart were in love.

FOLKLORE AND USAGE

❀ In China, bleeding heart was traditionally used as a love oracle by crushing the flower and observing the color of the juice. If it was red, then your love was returned; if it was white, then your love was in vain.

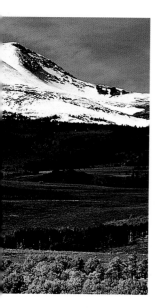

ABOVE *Bleeding heart grows wild in the Sierra Nevada mountains in North America, flowering from May to July.*

Key words
POSITIVE: *Emotional freedom, detachment, unconditional love.*
NEGATIVE: *Possessiveness, emotional dependence, attachment.*

Challenge
To release the toxicity of unrecognized emotional neediness and to love with detachment.

CASE STUDY

Paula, a 49-year-old woman, was seeking a divorce because she felt emotionally unfulfilled in her marriage.
She complained that her husband didn't understand her, was always working, and never gave her enough affection. She thought he needed to see a counselor to overcome his coldness. He felt that the marriage was a good one and didn't want to break it up and agreed to go with her to marriage guidance.

Outside the counselor's house there were several Bleeding Heart plants that Paula felt very drawn to. She was given the essence and during counseling she discovered to her surprise that, far from feeling cold toward her, her husband was reacting to her needy emotional dependency. She wept a lot about her childhood, which had been abusive, and saw how she was expecting her husband to make up for her parental neglect. She was expecting the counseling to confirm her belief that it would be better to divorce, but to her surprise as the counseling continued, she found a new, more balanced partnership with her husband.

BECOME EMOTIONALLY DETACHED

ENABLES YOU TO STAND ALONE

RIGHT *Bleeding Heart flower essence will help you to achieve emotional detachment and independence.*

Therapeutic actions
Purifies overattachment and dependency; brings strength and integrity to love relationships.

Method of making essence
Sun method.

Ways of using and use in combination
Very good with Walnut and Chicory; make it into a lotion with Dandelion and rub around your heart area.

Best supportive technique
Write the story of your heart, from as far back as you can remember. Show it to a trusted friend or therapist for comment. Keep a journal to gain some objectivity.

Epilobium angustifolium

Fireweed

CALLED WILLOWHERB *or rosebay willowherb in Europe, fireweed is from the* Onagracea *family, which contains the wonderful evening primrose and the fuchsia. The most varied gathering of this family is in the United States but* Epilobium angustifolium *is a true native to both sides of the Atlantic. It is a survivor of the days before the land bridge between Alaska and Siberia vanished beneath the ocean. It not only provides human medicine but also brings healing grace to the land itself.*

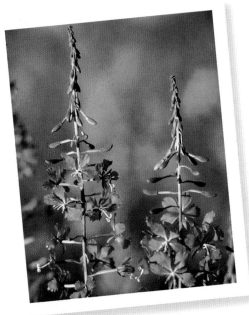

ABOVE *The flowers of the fireweed, which are borne on tall stems, are either white or a magnificent magenta-pink.*

SIGNATURE

❧ *Bravely renew life after total devastation* ❧

Name
It is also known as rosebay, willowherb, and bombweed. *Epilobium* **comes from** *epi,* **upon and** *lobos,* **a pod.** *Angustifolium* **means narrow-leaved.**

Color/shape
Fireweed flowers are borne in spires on tall stems; the single blossoms, about 0.75in. (2cm) across, have the texture of poppies and are rich magenta-pink or white. Each blossom consists of four magenta petals. Magenta is the color of the highest healing energy that emanates from just above our heads, while the number four represents the energy that grounds us into the physical realm. So fireweed brings the highest healing energy into physical being.

The lower lilac-purple blossoms open first, moving up the stem to reveal a continuous show of radiant color – an image of the dedicated energy needed to face and deal with, and eventually to transcend, devastation. After blooming, long pods are formed. At maturity, the pods split open and release downy fluff that is blown far and wide to new ground.

Habitat and growth pattern
Fireweed likes to re-vegetate waste ground. After forest fires and clearings, seeds that have been lying dormant for years emerge and take advantage of the added sunlight. It grew abundantly in the rubble of bomb sites all over Britain after World War II, giving colorful cheer to the survivors.

Fireweed proliferates by self-sown seedlings and running rootstock. It is one of the few wild flowers to be increasing in population because of urbanization. It is a great survivor itself.

FOLKLORE AND USAGE

❀ The great 15th century herbalist Gerard called fireweed "brave flowers of great beautie."

❀ At one time, stockings were woven from a mixture of cotton and the down from the seeds. In this way, fireweed can be physically as well as vibrationally protective.

NOTES

Therapeutic actions
Cleanses old patterns from the body and stimulates renewal of energies on all levels of being; attracts restorative healing energy from our surroundings.

Method of making essence
Sun method.

Ways of using and use in combination
Use in emergencies to release pain, trauma, and discomfort from the body and mind; water or spray unhealthy plants with a few drops of Fireweed essence in a pint of water.

Best supportive technique
Be in close contact with nature and become aware of its enormous regenerative powers. Grow something!

BELOW *A few drops of Fireweed essence will help to keep your plants healthy.*

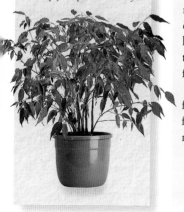

Key words
POSITIVE: *Survival, bravery, transformation, healing.*
NEGATIVE: *Devastation.*

Challenge
To face old injuries and utilize with faith the healing power of nature.

AFFIRMATION
I rise, like a phoenix from the ashes.

RIGHT *Fireweed is a great survivor, and during World War II it was one of the first plants to grow on the sites of bombed out buildings.*

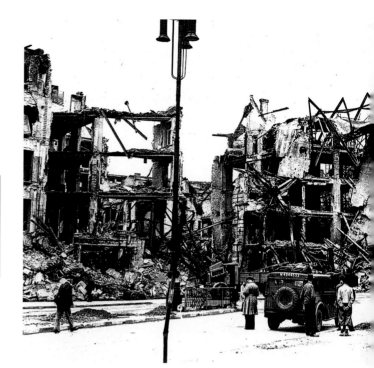

CASE STUDY

Joyce is in her 60s. She came to flower essence therapy because she suffered from chronic fatigue syndrome.
Her husband had suffered from severe financial loss due to the economic depression. This had forced them to move many times. Joyce felt devastated after each move and felt devoid of energy. She felt she would rather die than have to carry on supporting herself and her husband through their worsening financial situation.

After taking Fireweed for only a week, Joyce found that she was able to rest more deeply and felt replenished. Her mood lifted and she began to feel more hopeful about her health improving. The other therapies she was working with all seemed to have more effect. She enjoyed learning about the flower essences and found she had a real talent for prescribing them. She renewed her creative role in her family and made new friendships in the area, gradually finding the strength to pick up the threads of her life again.

RIGHT *Constant moving left Joyce with little energy until she discovered the healing benefits of Fireweed.*

Eucalyptus caesis

Silver Princess

THE EUCALYPTUS *family is closely associated with Australia. Threequarters of all the forest trees of Australia are eucalypts. There are over 500 species of these "gum trees." Their evergreen beauty dominates all but the driest places of Australia, growing from the snowline through to the central desert.*

They also grow in the Philippines, Malaysia, Indonesia, Papua New Guinea, and Melanesia where they are widely cultivated for their timber, spices, essential oils, edible fruits, and for their ornamental value. Although it is a subtropical tree, eucalyptus is now grown in the warmer parts of Europe for its usefulness and attractiveness. Eucalyptus was cultivated in California in the 1880s as a cure for malaria. The eucalypt flowers are composed of large skirts of white, creamy yellow, or red stamens.

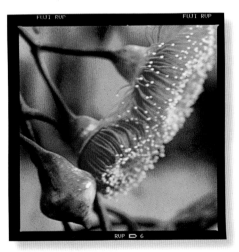

ABOVE *The flowers are deep red, the color of energy and action.*

SIGNATURE

❦ *Renew positive energy to overcome all obstacles* ❧

Name
It is also called ironbark. In Greek, *eu* means well, and *kalyptos* means cover, referring to the conical cap that fits tightly over the buds. *Caesius* means bluish or grayish green, the color of the bark.

Color/shape
The small, hard, white bell-shaped cap over the buds is a fusion of sepals. It is strong and holds the flowers tight inside. The flowers have no petals, only stamens, which means there is a complete concentration of energy. The cap is pushed off by the powerful growth of these stamens that emerge to dangle on long stems of swaying branches. Each flower is up to 1.5in. (4cm) across. They are deep pink-red, with a fringe of firm stamens around the large, light-yellow style. When the conical cap falls off, it is amazing to see how much beauty and energy has been trapped inside – all that hidden potential awaiting for the time to express itself.

Habitat and growth pattern
The branches of the eucalyptus droop down almost to the ground. This eucalypt is rare and grows only in the wild, on ancient granite outcrops of the wheat belt of the southwest of Western Australia. It has adapted to poor soil and extremes of temperature. The branches are snow-white because of the powder that covers them. This reflects the dry heat and traps some humidity on the surface.

The young trees bear semicircular leaves that clasp the stem in pairs, while the adult trees hang their slender leaves sideways on drooping twigs. The leaves are silver when young, turning blue-gray in color like the trunk. The buds, seed capsules, and young branches are also silvery. The general effect of silver is to help you move faster and communicate better – like quicksilver.

FOLKLORE AND USAGE

✿ Although it is *Eucalyptus globulus* that is most commonly used commercially, the leaves of all the eucalypts make a very useful aromatic oil that is both fresh and stimulating. It is anti-bacterial and effective in inhalations and for muscular fatigue.

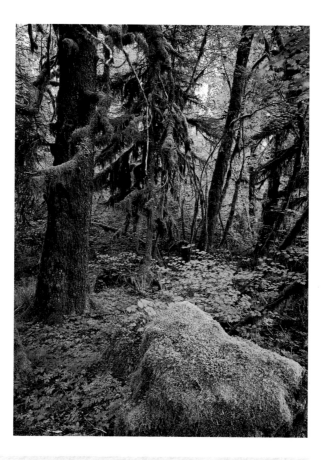

AFFIRMATION
I free myself from the past and take actions that reflect my life purpose.

Key words
POSITIVE: *Motivation, enthusiasm, purpose.*
NEGATIVE: *Aimless, despondent, rebellious, frustrated.*

Challenge
To release the past and formulate goals that inspire joy.

RIGHT *More than 75 percent of the trees in the Australian forests belong to the eucalyptus family.*

James, a 30-year-old computer programmer, was usually a very lively and curious person interested in the arts and sciences.
He was successful enough in his job, but for several months he had been very depressed, creating conflict with his colleagues. He was very frustrated, flat, and exhausted as a result, and didn't know what to do with himself.

After taking Silver Princess for a week, James realized that he felt his life wasn't going anywhere. Two weeks later he realized that he'd started moving in potentially creative directions but none of them had brought the fulfilment that he needed. Holding on to past successes was holding him back and he needed a new goal. For a time he couldn't decide what that might be, but after another couple of weeks of taking Silver Princess, he made a decision to train in computer graphics. This would both satisfy his creativity and build on his previous experience. He felt immeasurably better and got back his zest for life.

NOTES

Therapeutic actions
Brings back motivation and the drive to fulfil life potential; helps in moving on to the next stage of growth when impetus is lacking.

Method of making essence
Sun method.

Ways of using and use in combination
Use twice daily in dosage bottle, night and morning. This essence needs to be taken for more than two weeks to feel its impact. Use on the Shenmen point

in the ear, dabbed on with a Q-tip. This is useful when someone is prevented from living a positive life because of addiction.

SHENMEN POINT

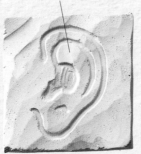

ABOVE *Apply the essence to the Shenmen point on the ear.*

Best supportive technique
Take time to answer the following questions:
What do I want from my life? How do I envisage my future? What would I be thinking, feeling, sensing, smelling, seeing if I were doing what I wanted? What obstacles do I envisage to this, and how can I overcome them? What would be the cost of this outcome?
If the cost is too great, go back and start again, reformulating your goals until you energize your own ability to conceptualize your future.

Fraxinus excelsior

Ash

ASH *is a member of the* Oleaceae *(olive) family.* Fraxinus excelsior *is the most common of the 65 different species. It is a large forest tree native to Europe. It can grow up to 80ft. (25m). Because ash trees come into leaf after other trees, and because they can live as long as 300 years, they are taken to represent maturity and growing strength.*

BELOW *The black bud and paired leaflets look like the traditional hooded figure of death with outstretched arms.*

LEFT *Symbolic of maturity and strength, ash trees can live as long as 300 years.*

🌹 *The key to wise choice is to gain perspective* 🌹

Name
"Ash" comes from the Anglo-Saxon word *easc* **for the tree.** *Excelsior* **refers to its great height and width.**

Color/shape
Ash is a deciduous tree that bears conspicuous black buds in the winter. The black buds look like the traditional hooded figure of death, and indeed the tree is related to both birth and death. In the early spring, both male and female flowers appear before the leaves, either on the same or on separate trees. The greenish-yellow, greenish-white or reddish-purple flowers cluster densely together. The minute flowers have no petals or sepals. The abundant pollen is wind-borne so there is no need to attract insects for pollination. The flowers come early and pollinate while other trees are just beginning to show their leaves.

Habitat and growth pattern
Ash tree fruits are winged seeds, called "keys," produced by the female tree. After spreading far and wide, the seeds lie dormant for a full 18 months before sprouting.

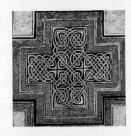

ABOVE *Ash represented the cycle of reincarnation to the Celts.*

The beautifully designed leaves are long and consist of 9 to 13 stalked leaflets that give the tree a light and graceful appearance. Being both fast-growing and easy to set seed, ash can be seen as an abundant creator of life. It is vigorous, dense-rooted, and demanding of the soil; it is easy to transplant but bad to grow near shrubs because it is liable to use all the nutrients in the soil for itself. Ash really knows how to get what it needs to survive and can live as long as 300 years.

The twisting stem echoes the turning "keys," and is reminiscent of the turns of the *caduceus* as it creates the chakra system along the spine. All these signatures mount up to a deep connection of the ash with birth, abundance, life, and death.

CASE STUDY

Sue is in her late 50s and has many family and care commitments. She was beginning to focus more on her own life and to find interests outside the home, so these commitments were causing her an increased feeling of restriction and resentment. When she began taking Ash, Sue found its effects uncomfortable at first, but she continued with the recommended use. She noticed few changes within herself, except that she was gradually becoming more assertive.

After a couple of weeks, family members seemed more tolerant of her wishes. When she looked more closely at what was happening, she saw that she was able to stand up for her own choices now in a way that didn't create friction. She supposed the initial discomfort with Ash essence was connected with getting used to standing up for herself and viewing the family dynamics in a more objective light. She had been able to stand back, take an overview of her life, and make wise decisions for her future happiness.

AFFIRMATION
I open my mind to my inherently spiritual nature.

Key words
POSITIVE: *Perspective, detachment, clarification of value.*
NEGATIVE: *Restriction, short-range vision.*

Challenge
To take a detached view of your life so that you can find values that are in harmony with your spiritual nature.

NOTES

Therapeutic actions
Helps to create a space of calm detachment, giving flexibility, adaptability, strength, a sense of what is real, and, sense of your true values.

Method of making essence
Boiling method.

Ways of using and use in combination
Dosage bottle and ointment.

Best supportive technique
Complete the following sentences: "When I die, I want people to say that I ..." "If I only had a year to live, then I would ..."

FOLKLORE AND USAGE

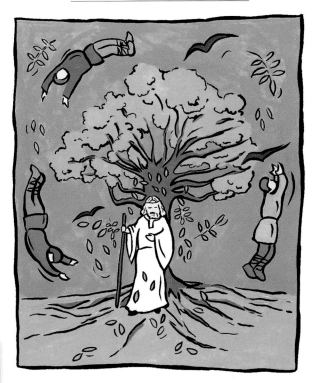

ABOVE *The ash tree is the Scandinavian World Tree, the central point of their world.*

❁ The ash is the World Tree – Yggdrasil of Scandinavian mythology. Its roots and branches bind together heaven and earth and hell, and at its root is a fountain of wonderful virtues. It is the tree of life and knowledge, and of time and space.

❁ To the Celts it represented the eternal round of birth and death and reincarnation.

❁ Ash twigs placed in a circle are a traditional protection against adders.

❁ Farm tools and implements were made of ash because the white lumber is strong and flexible and is able to bear more weight or impact than any other wood.

❁ The medicinal properties of ash bark have been used as a bitter tonic and astringent to treat fever and as a substitute for quinine. An infusion of the leaves is used to regulate bowel movements, to expel intestinal parasites, to reduce fever, and to alleviate rheumatic and gouty pains. The leaves are used externally in compresses or in bath preparations to treat suppurating wounds. It is a very useful, versatile, and flexible tree that can help us to be strong and flexible too.

Gardenia megasperma

Bush Gardenia

GARDENIA MEGASPERMA *belongs to the family of* Rubiaceae, *which is one of the largest flowering plant families. Most tropical species are evergreen trees or shrubs growing in open woodland or savanna in tropical regions of Africa, Asia, or Australia, while those growing in temperate regions, even including the Arctic and Antarctic, are herbaceous. The best-known European genera are the bedstraws and woodruff. Of tropical flowering shrubs in the family, gardenia is the most popular for ornamental purposes. This particular gardenia grows in the open woodland and tropical forests of the Northern Territory of Australia.*

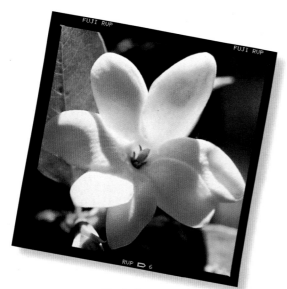

ABOVE *Gardenia megasperma has attractive white flowers, the color of grace, innocence, and love.*

SIGNATURE

The beautiful fragrance reminds us of the sweetness of relationships

Name
Gardenia is named after Dr. Alexander Garden, a Scottish physician and naturalist who lived in the United States. The word *megasperma* **comes from the Greek** *mega*, **meaning big, and** *sperma* , **which means seed.**

Color/shape
Gardenia is known for its gorgeous waxy-looking flowers that are reminiscent of roses but without the thorns. They have 5 to 11 petals and a wonderfully fragrant smell that has traditionally been connected with romance and love. This gardenia is white with nine petals. White is connected with innocence and grace, and the number nine represents near fulfilment of a plan, so it can be represented as bringing pure love to completion.

Habitat and growth pattern
Gardenia grows up to 30ft. (9m) high with a rounded crown and crooked branches. It blooms from July to November. The bark is smooth, mottled, yellowish, and powdery, which sets off the attractive foliage. The leaves are smooth and velvety when young, gradually becoming leathery. They are simple with a prominent herringbone vein.

The fruit is hard and contains many edible seeds, which are filled with a sweet, thick juice embedded in a pulpy material. This can be seen as representing the fruitfulness of relationships.

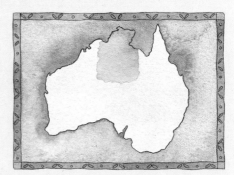

ABOVE *The bush gardenia is a native species of Australia's Northern Territory.*

AFFIRMATION
I create intimate relationships that fulfil my deepest desires.

Key words
POSITIVE: *Renewal of intimacy, improved communication.*
NEGATIVE: *Unaware family relationships, lack of intimacy, tactlessness.*

Challenge
To make time to communicate sensitively with loved ones.

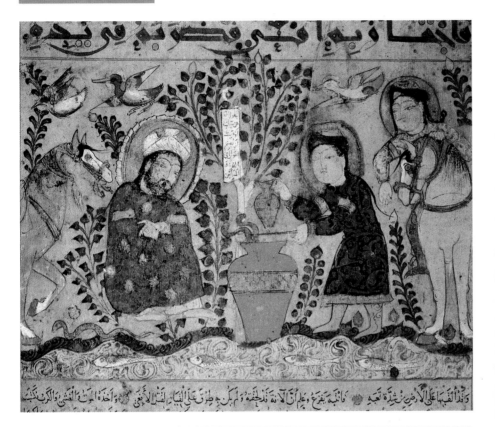

ABOVE *Gardenia has many uses in Chinese medicine, and is known as the happiness herb.*

FOLKLORE AND USAGE

❂ In Chinese herbalism, gardenia is used as an anti-inflammatory and is known as the happiness herb. It is believed to relieve liver congestion and blocked emotions. It also calms the heart. Not surprisingly, the essence opens up blocked feelings of intimacy, which calms and brings about emotional satisfaction.

NOTES

Therapeutic actions
Brings renewed interest in family relationships, especially with a spouse; brings an ability to relate more successfully to siblings, parents, children, or friends.

Method of making essence
Sun method.

Ways of using and use in combination
Dosage bottle, taken night and morning.

Best supportive technique
Read "Being Intimate – A Guide to Successful Relationships" by John and Kris Amodeo.
(See pp. 140–141).

Georgina came to flower essence therapy because she was feeling very depressed.
She and her husband both worked from home in the same office space. Although they worked well together, it was clear that Georgina felt restless and lonely because working so hard at home had taken all the fun out of their relationship. In the past they had come home at the end of the day to find comfort and amusement with each other, telling tales of what had happened during the day and planning carefully how they would spend their vacation time together.

Georgina was losing interest in her husband as a lover and was seeing him more as an office colleague. After taking Bush Gardenia, however, she began to be enthusiastic about spending time with him again.
They bought a shed to put in their large backyard where they could play table tennis. They also began to set aside time for telling each other their nightly dreams, and spent time each week renewing their sexual intimacy. Georgina's depression quickly vanished.

Geranium erianthum

Sticky Geranium

THE GERANIACEAE *family is small but is very common in temperate and subtropical regions of both the northern and southern hemispheres. It is, though, a very adaptable family since some grow even in the Arctic and the Antarctic. There are two branches to this family: the geraniums and the pelargoniums. The so-called geraniums grown so often in pots, yards, and greenhouses in fact belong to the group of pelargoniums from South Africa.*

SIGNATURE

❦ *Renewed power comes from energetic and wise action* ❦

Name
Geranium comes from *geranion*, **Greek for crane. This exciting little flower is a member of the cranesbill family, so called because their fruits are reminiscent of beaks.**

Color/shape
There are five leaflets that support five pinky-purple heart-shaped petals that have five long and five short stamens, all closely joined around the two sets of five styles and five graceful stigmas.

The petals are beautifully veined like fine ink lines and stand out because the texture is so delicate. The number five relates to our five senses, so it can be seen as being about coming to our senses.

Habitat and growth pattern
The geranium's seed pods split open as the mature fruit dries out, curling up and suddenly catapulting their seeds afar like ballistic missiles.

FOLKLORE AND USAGE

✸ The crane is associated with preserving and transmitting wisdom in the Celtic tradition. This is connected to the fact that the crane's flight was said to have inspired the Celtic ogham alphabet because of the pattern made by their long legs in flight. The crane stands on one leg close by the water and stoops down to catch fish with its long beak, never even getting wet. This can be seen symbolically as using insight to see through confusing emotions and pick out what is important to act on – a quality that the geranium can bring out in us.

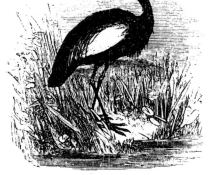

ABOVE *The sticky geranium is a member of the cranesbill family, so called because the fruit resembles a crane's beak.*

ABOVE *The sticky geranium flower has five petals, the same number as our senses, with which it is associated.*

Key words

POSITIVE: *Finding inner wisdom, getting unstuck.*

NEGATIVE: *Procrastination, lack of insight.*

Challenge

To see the self in a powerful light in order to release new potential.

NOTES

Therapeutic actions
Attunes you to your inner knowledge and empowers you to free up your inner potential to go beyond previous states of growth and self-definition.

Method of making essence
Sun method.

Ways of using and use in combination
Dosage bottle; with Walnut, Borage, and Thyme essences.

Best supportive technique
Imagine that the change you want to make has already happened – what does it feel like? Allow yourself to experience the positive feelings, thoughts, and sensations.

RIGHT *The crane in flight is said to have inspired the Celtic ogham alphabet.*

CASE STUDY

Philippa, age 40, is a talented artist but was frustrated because she never had enough time to devote to her work. She suffered from asthma that was also getting progressively worse. Philippa had had various commissions offered to her, but could not accept them because so much of her emotional and physical energy went into her parttime job in a restaurant. She felt powerless to change the situation, because the restaurant owner was her friend. She did not dare ask for more money for fear of causing offense and couldn't leave for fear of letting her friend down. She had been working there for six years and now felt unable to extricate herself from this draining situation. After taking Sticky Geranium for one month she realized how much of her potential was being wasted and gave in her notice. She began to devote more of her time to her art, which not only gave her increased insight into herself but also proved financially more rewarding too. Her asthma also began to get much better.

PHILIPPA'S ASTHMA IMPROVED

SHE FELT HER PHYSICAL ENERGY RETURNING

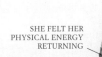

LEFT *Sticky Geranium helped Philippa to realize what was really important in her life.*

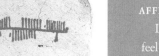

AFFIRMATION
I act and feel my power.

Helianthemum nummularium

Rock Rose

HELIANTHEMUM NUMMULARIUM *belongs to the* Cistaceae *or rock rose family, which like dry, sunny, rocky places such as in the Mediterranean and eastern United States, as well as enjoying warmer parts of Britain and Scandinavia. The hardy evergreen shrubs come into flower in the spring and often last until the fall. There are many hybrids that make very beautiful flowers for any garden, particularly in rock gardens since they thrive in open rocky areas. They have mostly large, ostentatious, short-lived flowers.*

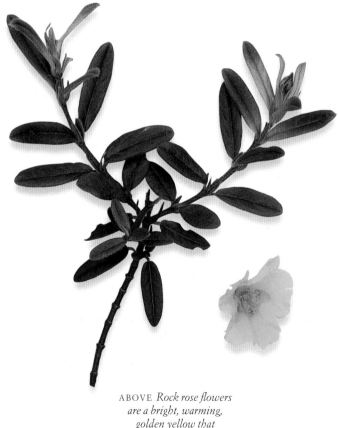

ABOVE *Rock rose flowers are a bright, warming, golden yellow that reminds us of sunshine.*

SIGNATURE

The Light of the Spirit liberates us from all fear and terror

Name
Helianthemum from Greek *helios* for sun, *anthemon* for flower; *nummularium* from *nummulus* for little pieces of money, hence *nummularium*, a place of little pieces of money.

Color/shape
The flowers are bright, sulfur yellow with numerous golden stamens in a tuft surrounding the pistil. They are five-petaled, flat, and open – radiant – like golden coins lying in the grass. Their yellow color stores heat from the sun, multiplying the sun's rays for all to be warmed.

The petals are crumpled like tissue paper and the flowers soon fade and die. The thin petals like to open in sunny weather and soon fall from the flower if they are gathered.

In wet weather and at night they close their petals. These facts tell us of their transitory nature, which contrasts with their bold color, as the fragile body contrasts with the eternal nature of the soul.

Habitat and growth pattern
Rock rose spreads its many branching woody stems close along the ground. Only when we are disconnected from our grounding can fear take us over. It likes open rocky places such as chalky cliffs and stony hillsides where the grass is short. When we feel connected to the earth with our attention in spirit we can face those challenges that have the power to rock us the most. The fact that it can self-pollinate by closing its petals up shows the power we can find inside us when we need to.

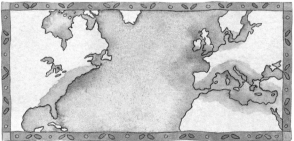

ABOVE *Rock rose grows in the Mediterranean, Scandinavia, Britain, and the United States.*

Key words

POSITIVE: *Courage, peace, and mental clarity.*
NEGATIVE: *Emergency, terror, panic, and extreme fear.*

Challenge

To know that the transcendent power of Spirit is present within us whatever threats exist to soul, mind, or body.

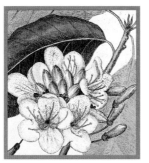

HELIANTHEMUM
NUMMULARIUM

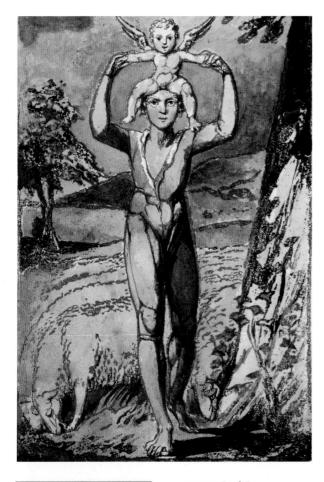

ABOVE *Rock Rose essence helps us to realize that we all have the transcendent power of the spirit within us.*

AFFIRMATION

The light of my spirit brings courage and endurance to face my challenge of…

CASE STUDY

Bernard had undergone a course of chemotherapy treatments for cancer that had resulted in extreme discomfort and sickness for many months.
He was feeling fairly strong before the side-effects of the treatments overtook him. Now he was severely weakened. He was grateful for his life having been saved but then another growth was discovered and he was recommended to take more chemotherapy. He was in deep shock and terror both with fear of death and of being unable to face another course of treatment with its devastating effects on his general health. He felt he would rather die than go through with the treatment and was at a loss what to do.

After taking Rock Rose Bernard found that he had the strength to postpone the chemotherapy treatment for a while and he began to explore other routes to health, including a strict diet and using what strength he had to live the life he really wanted to have.

NOTES

Therapeutic actions
Unfreezes terror and gives the courage to face the fear and take action. Gives a sense of the power in the transcendence of the human spirit.

Method of making essence
Sun method using only those plants that grow in the wild.

Ways of using and use in combination
Add other remedies as necessary, such as Walnut if you have the added burden of facing great change. Rock Rose is an important ingredient of Rescue Remedy or Five Flower Formula.

Best supportive technique
Ground in the senses, describing what you are physically seeing, hearing, or touching. Use the affirmation to clarify and identify the nature of your challenge exactly. Prayer, breathing, and the grounding techniques of polarity therapy, and various other exercises.

Helianthus annuus

Sunflower

HELIANTHUS ANNUUS *is the most magnificent of the sunflower or* Compositae *family. Of all the* Compositae*, it looks most like the sun – large with giant rays coming from it. The common sunflower is a large annual, native to western North America. It is both the Kansas state flower and the floral emblem of Peru. It also flourishes naturally in Mexico. It was cultivated by Native Americans some time before 1,000* B.C.E. *and was introduced to Europe in the 16th century. It became a major commercial food plant in Russia. It is now a popular plant the world over.*

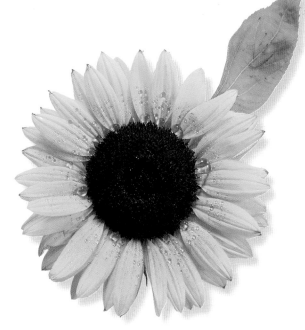

ABOVE *The statuesque sunflower can grow up to 10ft. (3m) high, with a flowerhead of 14in. (36cm).*

SIGNATURE

❧ *A balanced integration of the self* ❧

Name
Helios **means the sun and** *antheus* **a flower. It is called** *girasole* **in Italian, because it turns to face the sun.**

Color/shape
Sunflower heads are very large, as much as 14in. (36cm) in diameter. Brilliant yellow petals surround a yellow, orange, or brown flat central disk that is sometimes tinged red or purple. They bloom from July to September until the frosts begin.

The edible seeds form stunning geometric patterns, swirling both into and out from the center. The movement inward and the movement outward are balanced in an intricate wholeness.

Habitat and growth pattern
It is as though the sun has magnetized this great flower because it looks up at the sun even in the midday heat. At the end of the day it bows its head as if in humility to the earth, ready to be awoken the next day. In most societies, the sun represents the radiant positive male power of the cosmos, and the earth also represents the feminine as Mother Earth. The young sunflower roots itself strongly downward in the earth before reaching up to the sun, so it represents a balanced personality able to appreciate the polar opposites in the universe and in itself.

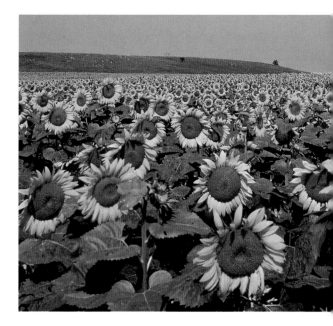

AFFIRMATION
My true sense of self grows as power and humility unite within me.

Key words
POSITIVE: *Integrated, balanced sense of self, humility.*
NEGATIVE: *Inadequacy, lack of self-esteem, over self-importance, arrogance.*

Challenge
To find the radiant self-esteem and generosity of your male energy.

BELOW *The sunflower is now grown all over the world as a crop.*

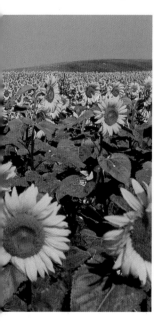

FOLKLORE AND USAGE

❉ Sunflowers have been highly valued by the indigenous people of America for at least 3,000 years. The stalks provided them with textile fiber, the leaves fodder, the flowers a yellow dye, and most important of all, the seeds provided food and hair oil. You can use all the parts of the sunflower.

❉ The Chinese have used the sunflower for thousands of years, and it was a sacred symbol in the ancient

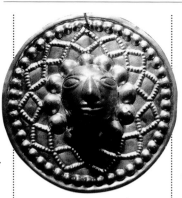

ABOVE *The Incas worshiped the sunflower as the earthly representative of the sun and wore gold jewelry with sunflower motifs.*

civilizations of Peru and Mexico. It was worshiped by the Incas as a symbol of the sun. During religious ceremonies the seeds were eaten and a large sunflower of pure gold adorned the breasts of the sun priestess.

❉ Sunflower is used to make paint, soap, cooking oil, and margarine.

❉ Sunflower oil contains a substance useful in the treatment of asthma.

NOTES

Therapeutic actions
Restores balance and wholeness to our sense of identity; nourishes the male aspect of the self in both men and women.

Method of making essence
Sun method.

Ways of using and use in combination
Universal remedy, can be used with benefit in many combinations, particularly Walnut and Larch.

Best supportive technique
Dreamwork; art therapy; attuning to the seasons; psychotherapy.

CASE STUDY

Jodie, in her late 30s, was suffering from depression. She had a good job as an office manager but did not get on well with the staff under her.
A few years earlier she had spent a lot of time, money, and energy training as an osteopath but dismissive remarks made to her by a senior male osteopath discouraged her from beginning her new career so she went back to office work where she felt a sense of importance.

As her story unfolded it was clear that, despite the forceful way she managed her role in the office, her lack of self-esteem was holding her back from her real vocation.

After taking Sunflower for a few weeks, she began to remember some enthusiastic and friendly encouragement given to her by another osteopath during her training. She had completely "forgotten" this earlier meeting. Gradually she began to feel a sense of worth. She began to become "less bossy" at the office and found that she enjoyed being kinder to her staff. She realized that she had always felt "either superior or inferior to others," but now she felt like "just another human being." Six months later she began her new career as an osteopath with real confidence.

Hypericum perforatum

St. John's Wort

HYPERICUM *is a branch of the larger family of* Guttiferae, *which is a group of trees and shrubs, many of which produce lumber, drugs, dyes, and fruits. Hypericum is widespread in temperate regions and in mountainous areas in the tropics. It is common in grassland, hedgerows, and open woods in Britain, especially on chalky soils.*

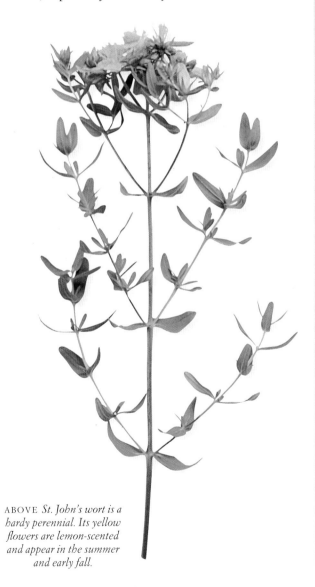

ABOVE *St. John's wort is a hardy perennial. Its yellow flowers are lemon-scented and appear in the summer and early fall.*

SIGNATURE

❧ *The outer sun is a source of inner strength* ❧

Name

Hypericum means "over a spirit" because it was used to drive away devils and evil spirits. *Perforatum* refers to the small translucent dots resembling punctures on the leaves, which are in fact oil glands. It is also known as Klamath weed because it naturalized around the Klamath River, California, at the beginning of this century. Its common name of St. John's wort refers to the fact that during the Crusades, the Knights of St. John of Jerusalem used it to heal the Crusaders' wounds.

Color/shape

St. John's wort flowers are very striking, 0.5–2in. (2–5cm) across, black dotted at the edge, with stamens in three bundles. The five yellow petals radiate outward, opening fully to the sun. The long stamens too expand into the space around them, like rays of light. The stem has two narrow wings running along its total length.

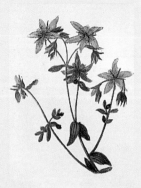

HYPERICUM PERFORATUM

This sun worshiper flower indicates that it would support those who are overexpanded; it is well able to help us to refocus as it matures to the earthy red color of the fruit. The red color is related to blood and to the contractive energy of the base chakra.

Habitat and growth pattern

St. John's wort is a spreading herbaceous perennial. It is fragrant and will thrive in most soils. Even though it is a great sun lover, it will tolerate light shade.

CASE STUDY

Judy, aged 35, was a television producer. She suffered from such bad nightmares that she was afraid to go to sleep at night. She feared that her son and daughter would be sexually abused and suspected people around her.

After taking St. John's Wort for just a week she had an experience of "a light going on in her head." She realized that she was seeing the "devil everywhere" because of her own past experiences of abuse. She was now able to talk about this for the first time and became more appropriately concerned for her own two children. Her nightmares stopped and she could sleep.

RIGHT Legend tells how St. Columba placed the St. John's wort flower under the head of a sleeping herdsman for protection.

AFFIRMATION
The sun is shining within me.

Key words
POSITIVE: *Contained inner light, strength.*
NEGATIVE: *Overexpansion, vulnerability, fear, disturbed dreams.*

Challenge
To experience the sun, not only as an outer reality but also as a source of inner strength and protection.

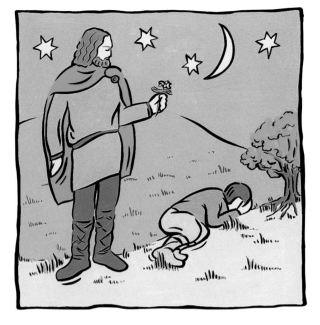

NOTES

Therapeutic actions
Internalizes the light-giving properties of the sun into the psyche; helps allergies and environmental stress, nightmares, night-sweating, bed-wetting; very effective for seasonal affective disorder.

Method of making essence
Sun method.

Ways of using and use in combination
Make an infusion by putting the flowers in olive oil until the oil turns deep red.

Best supportive technique
Make sure you get enough sunlight or natural light, at least 30 minutes a day, to nourish the pituitary gland.

FOLKLORE AND USAGE

❋ In Scotland the plant is dedicated to St. Columba. According to legend, Columba found his young cattle herder weeping because he was afraid that the cattle would stray during the night. Columba was said to have plucked the flower and put it under the child's arm, telling him to sleep in peace for no harm could then befall him.

❋ If St. John's wort was tied to a cradle, the child could never be ill-wished and was certain to thrive. In the folklore of the British Isles, stories abound about St. John's wort preserving the wearer from enchantment, the evil eye, and poisons.

❋ As well as its magical functions, St. John's wort was used medicinally to break up catarrh and congestion, for soothing and sedating, and as a remedy for melancholy and madness. When the blossoms are put in olive oil and left to infuse in the sun, the oil gradually becomes a beautiful rich red. This was known as St. John's blood and traditionally had remarkable healing properties.

❋ St. John's wort turns to follow the sun and blooms from June to August, but the height of its blossoming is at the Feast of St. John at the time of the summer solstice. It was used in solstice rites and rituals by the the Druids, the Celts, and the Saxons.

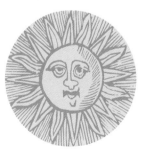

ABOVE St. John's wort was used at the summer solstice celebrations of the Druids.

Ilex aquifolium

Holly

BELONGING *to the* Aquifoliaceae *family, Holly was a major tree of the great primeval forests of Britain and central and southern Europe. It is also found in north Africa and west Asia and loves the moist soils of both the east and the Pacific coasts of the United States.*

BELOW *The holly bush has distinctive, tough leaves with spiny points.*

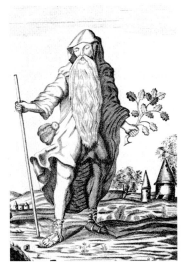

ABOVE *The Druids believe that holly guards against the evil spirits of the natural world.*

❦ *God's love protects us against our own negativity* ❧

Name
Christ's thorn or holy tree for its connection with Christ's passion. *Ilex* **is Latin for holm-oak.** *Aquifolium* **–** *aqua* **means water and** *folium* **means leaved, refering to the watery sheen on the holly plant's leaves.**

Color/shape
Holly blooms in May with male and female flowers appearing on separate trees. The female flower, which produces the holly berries after being pollinated by the male, is divided again into four sections forming another intricate equal armed cross. This indicates the need to balance the conflicting aspects of our human nature with love. The petal's outer color of pale pink softens the heart and the white inside speaks of purity.

Habitat and growth pattern
Holly is a much–branched evergreen needing little sun because its dark green shiny leaves reflect much light. The leaves have spiny points for protection. The leaves stay on the tree three to four years and even when they drop retain their strong form for some time. These give a sense of its warrior-like protection and security. In fact it is recommended by the police as more effective than barbed or electric wire to defend a house from invaders. The fruit too is very persistent, remaining on the tree all winter providing winter food for birds and wild animals, and holly leaves provide winter fodder for deer – images of its generosity.

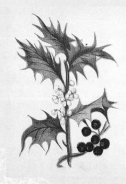

ILEX AQUIFOLIUM

Key words

POSITIVE: *Love, humility, and tolerance.*
NEGATIVE: *Hatred, jealousy, envy, suspicion, revenge.*

Challenge

To know that love is the primal force that created and sustains the universe and that it is always there for us.

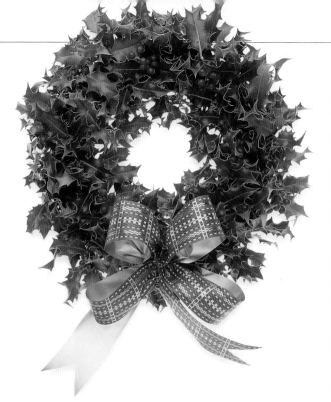

LEFT *To Christians, holly symbolizes the joy of Christmas as well as the crown of thorns.*

NOTES

Therapeutic actions
Releases and soothes strong negative emotions toward others. Brings a sense of love where it may have been seen as lacking. Protects us from our own negativity.

Method of making the essence
Boiling method. Male and/or female flowers can be used with a few leaves. Take twigs about 6in. (15cm) long.

Ways of using and use in combination
Dosage bottle, baths, ointments.

Best supportive technique
Any therapy or practice that opens up the heart. Trust yourself to loving and receiving love from whatever or whomever draws you.

CASE STUDY

Charlie, age five, had a new baby brother, Troy.
At first Charlie played happily with his brother. However, when Troy was only three months old Charlie began to squeeze Troy so tight that it made him cry. He would also pull his mother's hair when she was feeding Troy. When it was time for Charlie to go to school he would throw fierce tantrums and say he wanted to stay at home too. After taking Holly for a week his jealousy subsided and he went to school peacefully.

FOLKLORE AND USAGE

❊ It provided wood for the ancient Celts to make spear shafts, reputedly giving surety and balance to the thrower's aim. In mid-December the Romans gave holly as part of the five-day midwinter Saturnalia festival. To the Druids, holly guards us against all evil spirits, poisons, and the short-tempered or angry elementals of the nature kingdom.

❊ It represented Christ's Passion to the Christians because its thorny leaves and red berries symbolize the pain and blood that Christ endured for humanity.

❊ No Christmas scene is complete without the holly – the radiant round red berry contrasting with its prickly green leaves is a universal Western symbol of joy and goodwill during the hard times of winter.

RIGHT *The Romans gave holly as a gift during their Saturnalia midwinter festival.*

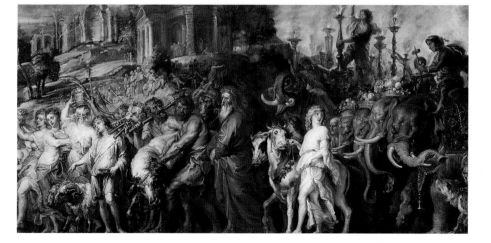

Impatiens glandulifera

Impatiens

IMPATIENS GLANDULIFERA *is a member of the* Balsaminaceae *or Balsam family and consists of about 850 species, mainly native to tropical Asia and Africa.* Impatiens *flowers are irregular in shape with five petals forming a broad lip, a hood, and curved spur behind. It is very different from the houseplant Busy Lizzie, also called* Impatiens. *Himalayan balsam, as it was named when it was brought from Kashmir to Britain in 1839, has naturalized along waterways and waste places.*

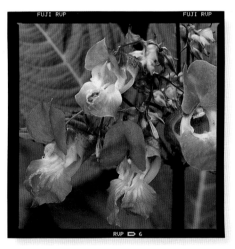

ABOVE *Impatiens has delicate pink flowers, each of which is composed of five petals.*

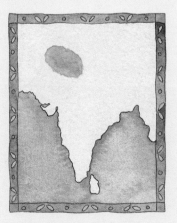

ABOVE *Impatiens originated in the mountainous Kashmir region of India.*

Key words

POSITIVE: *Cooperative, gentle, balanced poise.*
NEGATIVE: *Impatience leading to physical, emotional, or mental tension, and irritation.*

Challenge

To use inherent mental, physical, and emotional energy without violence to self or others.

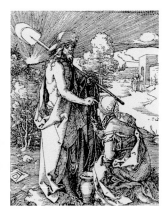

ABOVE *Jesus Christ told Mary Magdalene to "touch-me-not" after the Resurrection, giving the plant one of its common names.*

FOLKLORE AND USAGE

❀ Monks used it to illustrate their herbals in medieval times because of its name – Noli-me-tangere, Latin for touch-me-not. St. John's Gospel reports that these were the words said by Christ to Mary Magdalene after the Resurrection.

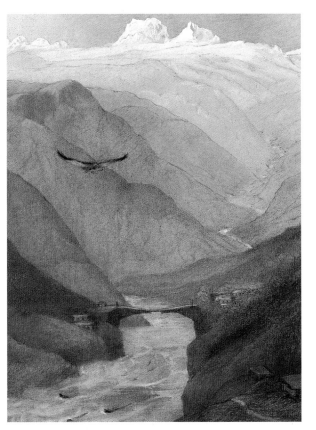

ABOVE *Impatiens essence helps you to relax and enables you to flow with the river of time.*

NOTES

Therapeutic actions
Increases acceptance of the natural flow of life and the pace of others. Releases tension from body, mind, and emotions where this is rooted in impatience.

Method of making essence
Sun method, using only the pale mauve kind. The hot mauve mottled with red will not do.

Ways of using and use in combination
Used in Rescue Remedy or Five Flower Formula. Combine with Dandelion to release physical aches and pains due to tension.

Best supportive technique
Deep breathing and conscious relaxation, as well as any relaxing physical activity such as polarity therapy exercises.

Jack is a very talented man, running his own small mail order business from home single-handedly.
He did an enormous amount of varied work each day, cursing himself if he didn't manage to send out the order the same day it arrived. When he wanted secretarial help he would do so very reluctantly because "they were so slow." He vowed to learn to type himself so that he wouldn't have to employ "slow coaches."

Gradually his already chronic backache worsened and he started to get swollen ankles. After taking Impatiens for a month he found that he was able to pace himself better and was happy to chat to temporary staff whose company he began to enjoy. He realized that he didn't always have to race against the clock and that his work time could be threaded with moments of relaxation and sociability. His back and his ankles were much improved.

Juglans regia

Walnut

WALNUT *belongs to the* Juglandaceae *family, which also includes hickories and pecans. Walnuts are deciduous trees that were widely cultivated in classical times throughout the Mediterranean. They are native to China and were believed to have been brought via Persia to Europe. This valuable nut and timber tree was taken north of the Alps by the conquering Roman legions.*

The white walnut, Juglans cinerea, *grows in the northern part of the United States and the American walnut,* Juglans nigra, *grows over a large area in the central and eastern states. The European walnut* Juglans regia *is widely cultivated in California, Australia, and all temperate countries for its nuts. It is also used both internally and externally as medicine.*

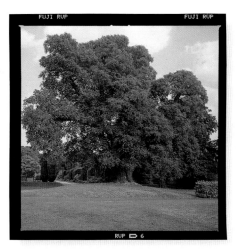

ABOVE *The walnut tree is slow-growing but can reach a height of 100ft. (30m) and live up to 300 years.*

NOTES

Therapeutic actions
Eases difficult transitions; releases negative influences preventing change; protects during important life transitions, such as teething, puberty, menopause; engages the will to move forward to the greater benefit of the mind, body, and spirit.

Method of making essence
Boiling method. Collect female flowers from several different trees.

Ways of using and use in combination
Use as a dosage bottle; can be used in most combinations about change to support other essences to do their work; can be made into an ointment and gently rubbed around the eyes to relieve change-induced stress.

Best supportive technique
Use well-founded conditions for change from neurolinguistic programing; get plenty of good food, sleep, and exercise; eat walnuts.

Key words
POSITIVE: *Protection during transition, skillful change toward true goals.*
NEGATIVE: *Stressful change, resistance to change, major biological and physical life transitions.*

Challenge
To be willing to move unhindered to your next stage of growth.

AFFIRMATION
I have all the protection I need to re-create my life according to my own personal ideals.

FOLKLORE AND USAGE

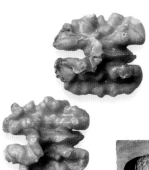

ABOVE *The walnut kernel is uncannily similar to the shape of the human brain, with left and right hemispheres.*

RIGHT *Walnuts were traditionally served at weddings in Ancient Rome to symbolize new beginnings.*

❀ The Roman emperor Marcus Aurelius Probus ordered wine shops to offer walnuts free of charge with wine to prevent drunkenness among his soldiers.

❀ The nuts were traditionally served at ancient Greek and Roman weddings.

❀ Walnut lumber is known for its beautiful grain, its strength and endurance.

❀ The leaves and the nuts are stringent and clean the intestines. It was also used to treat skin diseases. Culpeper suggested that "the distilled water of the green leaves cures foul running ulcers and sores." The thick peel around the nut contains vitamin C and can be used to seal up wounds. Wearing walnut leaves around the head can help to prevent headache and sunstroke.

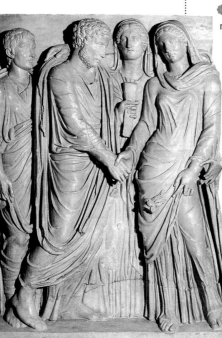

CASE STUDY

Eight year-old June had recently moved to a new house and changed schools. Very soon she was away from school with a racking whooping cough that persisted for five weeks. No medicine from the doctor or the homeopath seemed to to stop the awful cough. Her mother gave up her job for a time to nurse her, but this didn't seem to make any difference, so she returned to work, leaving June in the care of an old friend. June's mother decided to let her daughter have a dosage bottle of Walnut essence to see if that could help her. June really liked the little dropper bottle that contained the Walnut remedy, and because it was kept by her bedside she sipped it frequently, finishing the whole dosage bottle by the end of the first afternoon. When her mother returned from work, she found June's nose and eyes were streaming with cold. This persisted for two days, but that was the last of the whooping cough. June seemed much stronger emotionally and mentally to those around her and returned happily to school the next week.

Larix decidua

Larch

LARCH *is a distinctive member of the ancient pine family. It lives in the Alps and also thrives in the cool, mountainous regions north of the Arctic Circle. Elsewhere it is a lowland tree, growing in coniferous forests across the northern hemisphere. It was introduced into England in the early 17th century for ship-building. Although European in origin, it was widely planted for its high-quality wood in the upland areas of north-eastern United States, where it is now the most common larch.*

BELOW *The larch is fast-growing, but relatively short-lived. It loses its foliage in the fall.*

SIGNATURE

❧ *Unfulfilled potential realized* ❧

Name
Larix was the name given to pine resin, while *decidua* (deciduous) means that the leaves drop in the fall.

Color/shape
There is an air of defeat in the way that the larch branches droop down; even the slender top of the trunk curves gracefully, as if unable to hold itself erect. The outline is not like the crisp Christmas-tree shape of many of its relatives, although when full-grown it has a slim conical shape. It spreads its branches unpredictably and untidily. Its branches look slim and delicate, but in fact it can survive in the extremes of high altitudes. It can quickly grow up to 150ft. (45m) in height. The larch is full of potential strength, but does not reveal it.

Habitat and growth pattern
Larch is the only conifer that loses its leaves in the fall, so appearing weaker. But it is actually much stronger than most trees. The male "flowers" are yellow and the females are red, both growing and drooping on weak shoots. Larch needles are soft because, unlike other conifers, they are designed to last only one season. This apparent softness is part of a strong transformation process.

The larch needles give the tree a coarse, lumpy appearance and the branches droop. The cones often remain on the tree for several years after they mature – like the adolescent who is physically able to leave home but hasn't quite got the confidence.

The young trees establish themselves readily and soon grow very fast, six times faster than oak, and therefore larch has become a symbol for boldness. They are often used to protect slower growing and less hardy kinds of trees. Although it grows quickly and untidily, it is able to protect younger "siblings," like many adolescents do.

Key words
POSITIVE: *Self-confidence, self-expression.*
NEGATIVE: *Unexpressed potential, expectation of failure.*

Challenge
To understand that you may have potential for success as yet unrecognized by yourself or anyone else.

FOLKLORE AND USAGE

❉ The Roman emperor Augustus used larch wood for building the Forum in Rome. It was also used for building inside castles.

❉ Larch wood is tougher, stronger, and more durable than any other conifer except for yew.

❉ It is used in mining operations because it is able to resist worm attacks.

❉ Larch resin makes a good varnish.

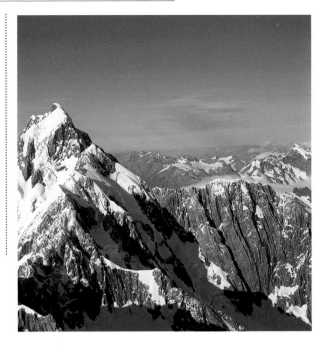

RIGHT *Native to the Alps, the larch tree also grows in the lowland areas of the northern hemisphere.*

CASE STUDY

Roberta, age 19, suffered from panic attacks. She was studying engineering at university but found it really boring.
After taking Larch for two weeks she realized that she was studying to please her parents. She gradually began to feel that she would like to be an actress although she had never done anything but school plays. After another month of taking Larch, she decided to leave university and join an acting class at the local college. She began enjoying her life and the panic attacks stopped. Roberta is now a drama teacher.

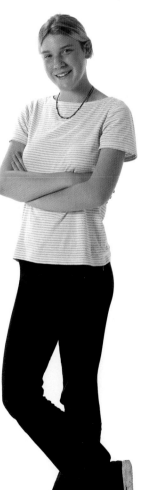

LEFT *Larch essence can help teenagers to grow in confidence and face those difficult adolescent years.*

NOTES

Therapeutic actions
Larch is a confidence-builder; brings awareness of potential for success and happiness; and increases self-esteem.

Method of making essence
Boiling method. In late March or early April pick twigs about 6in. (15cm) long, with some fresh young leaves and both male and female flowers. Use as many different trees as you can.

Ways of using and use in combination
Use in almost any combination to support self-esteem; use a dosage bottle; make into a lotion or compress to use around the diaphragm and/or throat.

Best supportive technique
Turn your hand to anything you choose, without worrying about failure; adapt the affirmation to say exactly what you want to achieve. Refer to Affirmations (see p.122) to ascertain what might be undermining you.

Lunaria annua

Honesty

T HE CRUCIFER *family grows as annuals, biennials, and perennials in disturbed ground, uncultivated fields, and woodland all over Europe and western Asia. Most vegetable crops of Europe and Asia are from this species – cabbages, Brussels sprouts, cauliflowers, various seed crops for oil, all belong to this industrious family. Lunaria annua is a relatively exotic member; its flowers are valued for their beautiful purple flower crosses in formal garden borders and for their satiny seed pods, which look attractive in dried flower arrangements.*

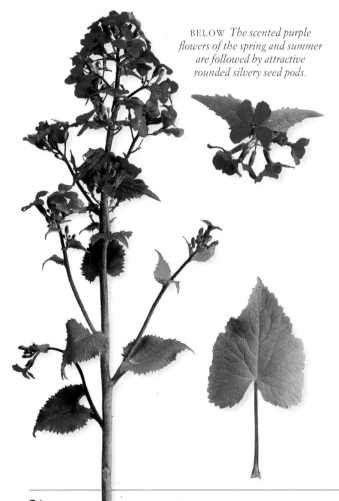

BELOW *The scented purple flowers of the spring and summer are followed by attractive rounded silvery seed pods.*

❦ *Be willing to suffer materially for higher values* ❧

Name

It is also called lunary, moneyplant, money-in-both-pockets, satinflower, or moonwort in the Britain and silver dollar or Peter's penny in the United States. *Lunaria* refers to the moon, and *annua* means annual. In Dutch it is *Judaspenning*, Judas's money, which indicates that it has to do with the betrayal of spiritual values. Its common name, honesty, is about rectifying this. The plant's family name *Crucifer* refers to the cross made by the four petals and four supporting sepals. *Crucio* can also mean torment.

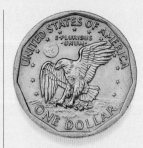

ABOVE *In the United States, honesty is also known as the silver dollar.*

ABOVE *Honesty is known as the moneyplant in Britain.*

Color/shape

The flowers make a shimmering pattern of purple or pink crosses. Almost all cruciform plants have white or yellow blossoms. This has a color similar to a bishop's cope.

Purple is connected with religious life in the language of symbolism.

Honesty's great circles of flat silvery seed vessels are like the moon or silver coins, and their inner covering is satiny, like mother-of-pearl.

The circle of the seed vessels relates to completeness, and the square formed by the cross of petals is connected with practicality. So honesty is a flower of practical spirituality with a beautiful silver lining.

The leaves are heart-shaped and toothed; this reminds us of the importance of protecting the heart.

Habitat and growth pattern

Honesty's flat seeds are easily dispersed by the wind, so the plant can seed very freely and generously. It is widespread on waste ground around human habitation.

NOTES

Therapeutic actions
Helps you to realize that nourishing yourself spiritually can bring healing to your physical body; good for the materialist or those who are obsessed with money worries; helps to integrate spiritual and material values; good for those who make the excuse that they don't have time for attending to their spiritual needs, and also for those who give and need acknowledgment – it helps them see, with gratitude, that they too are receiving the blessing of the divine giver within.

Method of making essence
Sun method.

Ways of using and use in combination
Dosage bottle; baths; good with Mullein.

Best supportive technique
Learn a meditation or prayer technique that suits you.

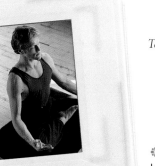

RIGHT *Meditation is an ideal supportive technique to use with Honesty essence.*

ABOVE *Honesty is sometimes grown solely for its attractive silvery seed pods.*

AFFIRMATION
I relate to the material world with integrity.

Key words
POSITIVE: *Spiritual life, detached giving.*
NEGATIVE: *Materialism.*

Challenge
To give and receive, knowing that the bounty of divine providence will flow.

FOLKLORE AND USAGE

❖ Honesty was traditionally believed to be able to put monsters to flight.

CASE STUDY

Jill was a social worker who felt burned-out from giving, so decided to turn her interior decorating hobby into a business. She was offered a contract unexpectedly and got excited about making the change – so excited that she gave an estimate that undervalued both her skills and the size of the job. She also found the work far harder than she had expected because she was continually having to adapt to her clients' demands. She argued with herself that she was lucky to get a break so soon into a new career, but she began to sleep badly and soon became seriously exhausted.

After taking Honesty for a couple of weeks, Jill began to realize that she had not really appreciated the value of her former job. The money that she earned from decorating was not enough to compensate her for the job satisfaction she'd once had. She missed helping others and saw that if she could become more detached, she would probably not get so bogged down. She tackled her clients and told them that they had to stop changing their minds and charged them for the extra work she had done.

After six months she went back to social work on a parttime contract basis. She felt more detached and consequently became less entangled in others' difficulties. Her sleep improved and she was able to take time out for herself for quiet periods. She was happy realizing her potential for giving.

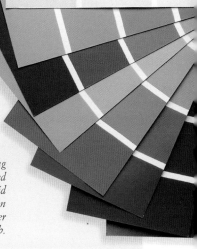

RIGHT *After taking honesty essence Jill realized that interior decorating did not give her job satisfaction and she returned to her former job.*

Macrophidia fuliginosa

Black Kangaroo Paw

THIS REMARKABLE *flower belongs to a larger kangaroo paw* (Haemodoracea) *family. A near relative,* Anigozanthos manglesii, *has the capacity to change to a wide variety of colors, such as red and green, purple and red, lilac, purple, or yellow, with no apparent biological, genetic, or chemical reason. Black kangaroo paw, however, is not so flexible. It differs from other kangaroo paws in the structure of the flower, which is more deeply and evenly divided. The three seeds of the fruit fall away, taking with them pieces of the base of the flower, but leaving the flower itself clinging persistently to the stem.*

A typical Australian plant, it grows in tropical climates in open ground at the edges of scrub.

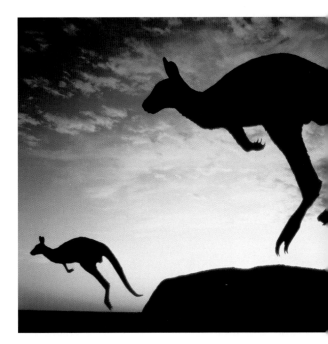

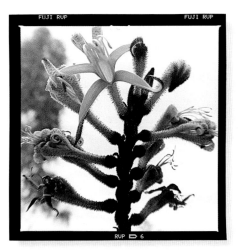

ABOVE *The yellow, tubular flowers of the black kangaroo plant are segmented into fingerlike sections.*

SIGNATURE

❧ *Transforms emotions from dark to light* ❧

Name
Macrophidia **is a corruption of** *Macropodia,* **the Latin name for the kangaroo;** *fuliginosa* **refers to the sooty appearance of the flowers and stalks.**

Color/shape
Black kangaroo paw grows in sprays of yellow, woolly, swollen, tubular flowers. The flowers are sharply segmented into fingers nearly 2in. (5cm) long, like kangaroo feet – each covered with black hairs. The fingers wave freely in the wind.

Habitat and growth pattern
The stout branched stems, which are also covered with black hair, grow to over 3ft. (1m). Each spring, fan-shaped tufts of narrow, sword-like, bluish-green leaves grow to 1ft. (30cm) alongside the sprays of flowers. The sword shape is traditionally associated with clarity of thought and fairness.

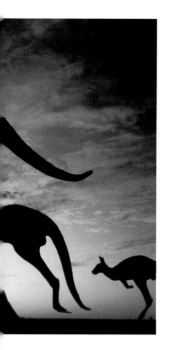

Key words

POSITIVE: *Love and forgiveness.*
NEGATIVE: *Hatred and revenge.*

Challenge

Become aware of and challenge the dark side of your nature so that you can transform hate into love.

LEFT *As the name suggests, the flowers of the black kangaroo paw species look like kangaroo feet.*

NOTES

Therapeutic actions
Encourages feelings of love and forgiveness that enable us to cut through powerful and obsessive negative emotions such as revenge, hatred, and the desire to dominate other people.

Method of making essence
Sun method.

Ways of using and use in combination
In a dosage bottle; rub into the upper back where there may be tension knots.

Best supportive technique
Talk to and confide in a trusted friend or therapist about the nature of your obsessions; know the power of love that hides within the passion of hatred; prayer and/or meditation.

AFFIRMATION
I take responsibility for my emotions and act from my better nature.

CASE STUDY

Derek came to counseling because he was going through an extremely painful and bitter divorce.
Although he had initiated the proceedings, believing that he would be happier with another woman, when he discovered that his wife was seeing another man he grew extremely jealous. He hadn't realized how attached he still was to her and became obsessive about her behavior, following her around and making angry scenes whenever they met. However, after a month of taking Black Kangaroo Paw at his counselor's suggestion, Derek came to his senses and realized how unproductive and harmful his behavior had been. He began to understand his reasons for wanting the divorce. He remembered how he had struggled to be happy with her for many years and how both of them had endured an enormous amount of misery and suffering in their marriage. He began to grieve for the loss of many years in struggling to make this relationship work and left his ex-wife alone to get on with her life.

MUSCLES MAY BECOME KNOTTED

TENSION IN THE SHOULDERS AND NECK

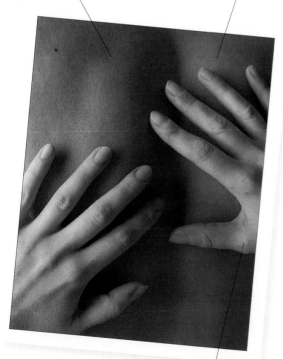

ABOVE *Black Kangaroo Paw may be rubbed on the back to soothe aches and pains, and release tension.*

RUB BLACK KANGAROO PAW ESSENCE ONTO BACK TO RELEASE TENSION

Macrozamia reidleii

Macrozamia

THIS REMARKABLE *plant belongs to the Zamiacea family. They are cycads, very ancient plants dating back 250 million years to Gondwanaland, which formed one of the huge landmasses before it broke up into separate continents. The macrozamia are a group of 12 species of cycads that look like ferns or small trees. They like open forest sites in southwest Australia and being in well-drained soil.*

SIGNATURE

Brings a balance of vitality for sexual healing

Name
Macrozamia **means a large Zamia. Pliny thought that the cones look very withered and named them** *Zamia* **which is Latin for loss.** *Reidleii* **is after the 18th-century French horticulturalist, Anselme Riedlei, who discovered the plant.**

Color/shape
Each plant has many fronds, like a palm growing from a base, and the male and female inflorescences or cones grow among the leaves.

Habitat and growth pattern
The male and female flowers are produced by distinct and separate plants. The male plant has three to seven cones that protect its pollen sacks. The seeds though become exposed – the male organ stays protected most of the time but is in fact very vulnerable when active. The sperms from it are capable of movement – vitality. The female macrozamia bears one or two flowers or cones that grow up to 20in. (50cm) high and can weigh as much as 6lb. (14kg).

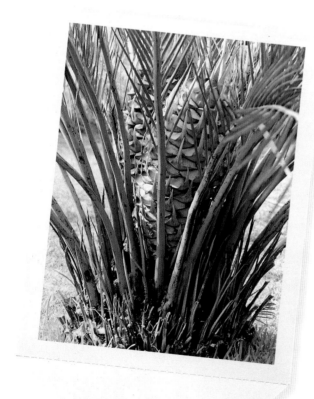

ABOVE *The distinctive cones of the macrozamia plant grow among tall palmlike fronds.*

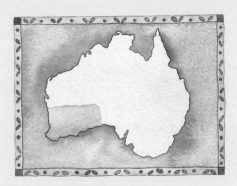

ABOVE *The Macrozamia species flourishes in the forests of southwest Australia.*

FOLKLORE AND USAGE

❀ A preparation made from the seed was used by the Aborigines of Australia for healing impotence. However, since the seed is highly toxic, this is not recommended.

❀ The light brown fluff that grows between the frond bases was used as a disposable diaper by aboriginal mothers.

CASE STUDY

Geraldine, a woman in her 40s, came to therapy because she hadn't been able to have sex with her husband for more than a year and was scared that he might leave her.

After taking Macrozamia for two weeks, she started to remember incidents connected to her sexuality. This included having a very abusive physician deliver her second child, which had left her with negative associations about her sexual organs. Other earlier memories surfaced that included inappropriate behavior from her father in her pubescent years. This included, among other things, leaving her unprotected with a trusted member of the community who sexually abused her. The accumulation of these painful associations had made her find the thought of sex repulsive. Taking Macrozamia helped bring these memories to her consciousness, and her counselor supported her in expressing her feelings. After a month of taking the essence she was able to be receptive again to her husband's advances.

NOTES

Therapeutic actions
Brings healing energy to all aspects of sexuality; heals people who have suffered or have made others suffer from incest, rape, or sexually inappropriate behavior; offers release from an over-preoccupation or aversion to sex; reduces sexual aggressiveness and promotes sensitivity. Through understanding the different functions of male and female, a healthy union can be achieved. The male can be free and vital and yet still learn from the protective and generous quality of the female.

Method of making essence
Sun and boiling method combined.

Ways of using and use in combination
Use in dosage bottle; make into a cream to massage into pelvic area; combine with Star of Bethlehem and self-heal for healing traumatic experiences.

Best supportive technique
Appropriate psychotherapy, such as a survivors' group or one-to-one psychotherapy.

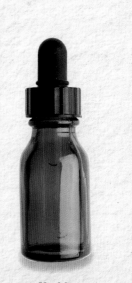

ABOVE *Use Macrozamia flower essence in dosage bottles to help heal sexual pain.*

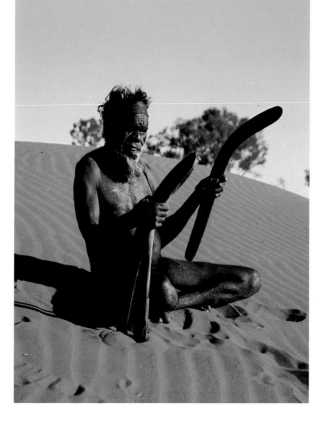

Key words
POSITIVE: *Sexual sensitivity and health.*
NEGATIVE: *Sexual abuse, domination.*

Challenge
Face the necessity of coming to a healing understanding of your sexual experience.

AFFIRMATION
As I sensitize myself to my own sexual healing, I find balance and personal fulfilment.

LEFT *Australian aborigines used the toxic seed of the macrozamia plant to make a potion to cure impotence.*

Madia elegans

Madia

MADIA *is a member of the tarweed group* (Madinnae), *which belongs to the* Asteraceae *branch of the sunflower family. There are many sticky-haired* madias, *such as pygmy madia, woodland madia, common hareleaf, and blow wives, which all grow in the Pacific states of the United States.* Madia elegans *is a native Californian wild flower that grows in the forest openings of the mountains.*

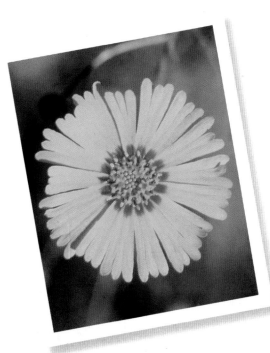

ABOVE *Madia looks like a target made of three rings – yellow, red, and a black honeycomb center.*

AFFIRMATION
I bring focus and clarity to every aspect of my life.

Key words
POSITIVE: *Clarity, enjoyment of detail, follow-through, enjoyable study.*
NEGATIVE: *Unfocused, scattered, can't concentrate.*

Challenge
To accomplish projects efficiently and thoroughly, to bring your spiritual goals into deeper focus.

NOTES

Therapeutic actions
Enables concentration, focus, and follow-through after action; helps combat feelings of lethargy when feeling overwhelmed by detailed work; helps us to discriminate; can bring into focus blocks to concentration that have been ignored.

Method of making essence
Sun method.

Ways of using and use in combination
Dosage bottle.

Best supportive technique
Practice a meditation technique every day.

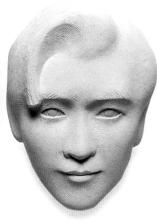

ABOVE *Use Madia essence as an aid to concentration. It will help to focus your mind on what is really important.*

CASE STUDY

Liz had been a natural student all her life. She had a curious mind and enjoyed exploring different topics from psychology to mathematics.

The problem was that she never finished anything, she got distracted and gave up or went on to another topic. She left university without finishing her degree, because she had never been able to complete assignments in her course work. As a 40-year-old, she continued to study but she still did not know what direction to go in. She had trained in secretarial skills, different sorts of counseling, and information technology, but she couldn't decide which way to go. Bach's Wild Oat helped her to decide to become a health practitioner but she still continued to be interested in everything and unable to complete anything.

Then she was given Madia, which immediately began to help her to focus on becoming a more proficient counselor. She began yet another counseling course, but this time she found she was able to overcome a lifetime's habit. Although at first she still tried to put too much information in her assignments, she managed to complete them. Gradually she was able to pinpoint themes and follow through ideas. Despite a lot of pressures in her home life, she used the course to organize her ideas and experiences from her previous training and completed it successfully.

Although she has learned how to focus and organize herself far better, Liz still needs to use Madia intensively from time to time.

BELOW *With the help of Madia essence, Liz began to learn how to focus her energies and stick to one thing at a time.*

MADIA HELPED HER TO CONCENTRATE ON ONE THING AT A TIME

LIZ STARTED TO ORGANIZE HERSELF MORE EFFICIENTLY

83

Malus sylvestris var. domestica

Apple

A MEMBER *of the* Rosaceae *family, apples are considered to be one of the oldest fruits used and cultivated by human beings, second only to the acorn. Around 2000* B.C.E. *an improved form of crab apple was developed,* Malus sylvestris var. domestica. *This apple tree is generally more graceful than its forebear the crab apple and the fruit is not bitter, but sweet. They look like super-fruits compared with the tiny crab apples. There are now an estimated 10,000 cultivated varieties of apples, some of which have been grown for hundreds of years. They cannot be grown successfully in tropical or subtropical regions because the trees have to experience temperatures below 45°F (7°C) before they will flower.*

BELOW *Apple blossom is renowned for its sweet and delicate scent.*

SIGNATURE

❧ *Through true knowledge, become whole* ❧

Name
Malus domestica **means a domesticated apple, and** *sylvestris* **means of the woods. The apple is truly domesticated because we have not only influenced the size, color, taste, and abundance of apples through cultivation, we have also modified the tree shape to make it accessible for picking.**

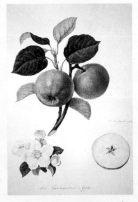

MALUS DOMESTICA

Color/shape
Apple flowers bloom in clusters of white or pink blossoms, each with five rounded petals. The fruit is spherical with an indentation at the core. It is 2–3.5in. (5–9cm) across with a sweet pulp. An apple cut across reveals that the pits are arranged in five-pointed stars, often with ten pit marks surrounding them. Five is the number of the planet Venus, the planet of love and beauty, and ten is the number of completion. Many myths surrounding the apple are based on this numerological fact.

Habitat and growth pattern
The crown of the tree is rounded and broad and can grow to a height of 40ft. (12m). There are many varieties of *Malus domestica*, **but generally the apple tree has a short trunk up to 2ft. (60cm) in diameter, often gnarled. The contrast between the gnarled tree and its crisp fresh blossom and fruit suggests the secret of youth that is contained in old age.**

BELOW *Apples are one of the most widely grown fruits for cooking and for eating raw.*

FOLKLORE AND USAGE

❋ Apples were sacred to Aphrodite, Venus, Hercules, Diana, Iduna, Dionysus, Olwen, Apollo, Hera, Athene, and Zeus.

❋ The stories and legends that involve eating apples, such as Adam and Eve, Snow White, and Fin McCool, are about radical transformation involving death and moving on to another state of being.

❋ In Greek myth, the apples of the Hesperides, which was similar to the Garden of Eden, are a symbol of the fruit of the spirit. In the myth, Hercules' 11th task symbolizes understanding the secret of transforming lust, anger, greed, attachment, and pride into continence, generosity, detachment, and humility. Although he found the magic apples, they were returned, because he couldn't master their secrets.

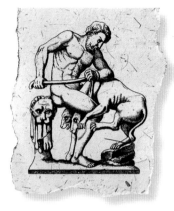

LEFT AND ABOVE *Apples feature in many myths of the ancient Greeks and Romans.*

❋ To Native Americans, the apple is a symbol of honor.

❋ The beautiful colors of the ripened fruit, which range from green to yellow to red, are another source of myth. Myth-makers saw this as suggesting that we have to make discerning choices about how we use our physical energy; we need to learn to use it wisely. For example, in the Greek myth of the judgment of Paris, the hero gave his hard-won golden apple to beautiful Aphrodite, rather than choosing the more ethical Hera, or the just Athene. Aphrodite, the goddess of love, then gave him the beautiful Helen. Since she was already married, this immature act of Paris started the bloody Trojan wars. So we mature by learning from our choices.

Key words
POSITIVE: *Convalescence, abundance of health.*
NEGATIVE: *Malingering illness, health-related fears.*

Challenge
To release unnecessary fears about health and know it as a natural state.

NOTES

Therapeutic actions
Reveals an understanding of the importance of health on all levels, physical, emotional, and spiritual; dissolves attitudes that prevent true healing; reduces fears about possible illness, such as catching infections, or genetic disposition to illness.

Method of making essence
Sun method.

Ways of using and use in combination
Use in the bath and in a dosage bottle; best used on its own.

Best supportive technique
Eat apples; if you are a woman, consider eating only apples one day a month, particularly just before menstruation.

CASE STUDY

Josephine had been ill with candidiasis for many years.
Although she was beginning to get well she remained anxious about her health. She began to eat apples regularly and take Apple essence. Soon she felt that good health was her natural state. This brought her great joy and she began to live a normal life again.

Malus sylvestris

Crab Apple

THE MALUS *family are deciduous trees and shrubs that grow in woodland and thickets throughout Europe, Asia, and North America. There are about 35 species of crab apple hybrids that are grown for their often fragrant flowers and attractive edible fruits.*

Fossil remains of apples have been found in Swiss Neolithic lake dwellings. Crab apples are believed to have recolonized the land after the end of the Ice Age. Malus sylvestris is the forerunner of many varieties of the eating apple, Malus x domestica.

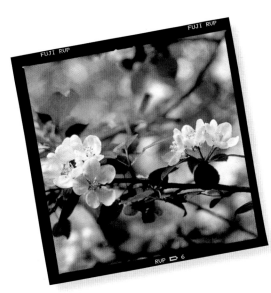

ABOVE *Crab apple blossom appears in late April or early May. It has a delicate fragrance.*

SIGNATURE

❧ *Balanced purification renews wholeness* ❧

Name
The common or wild crab apple gets its name from the Norse word *skrab*, which means a rough scrubby tree.

Color/shape
In the early spring, crab apple buds are blushed with pink, then in late April or May the lovely pale pink or white flowers bloom, a deep breath of purity after the dark winter, marking the edge of summer. These flowers are delightfully scented.

Crab apple flowers contrast with the thorny tree or shrub on which they grow, which has wrinkled bark and a knotted trunk. It is more like a bush than a tree, although it can grow to 30ft. (9m) high and 23ft. (7m) across. It is inelegant, old, and crabbed looking even when young. Its blue-gray bark flakes away, leaving brown patches. The opposites inherent in crab apple's signature are clear, the freshness and purity of the blossoms contrasting with the unkempt appearance of the tree. The tree likes light and space, often growing in small groups separately from other species of trees.

Habitat and growth pattern
The pink-flushed white flowers are followed by greenish-yellow, red-flushed fruit. They ripen by October to small, hard, golden apples with a yellow skin and a pale yellow flesh. The apples stay small and bitter. Cutting open the fruit reveals its close relationship to the domestic apple. The crab apple's membership of the rose family is clear from the flowers' five styles and stigmas.

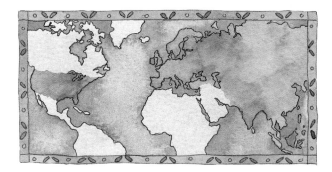

ABOVE *The Malus species can be found from North America to Asia.*

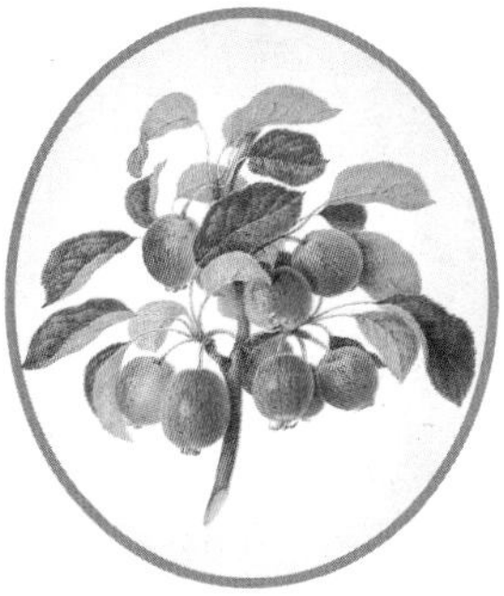

MALUS SYLVESTRIS

NOTES

Therapeutic actions
Brings a sense of inner purity; useful when fasting; restores a sense of balance to physical, emotional, or spiritual cleansing; heals a sense of shame or humiliation.

Method of making essence
Boiling method. Pick a whole cluster of flowers and leaves from the end twigs from several different trees.

Ways of using and use in combination
Use in baths and from a dosage bottle; use as a compress on an affected part; check whether you may need to use it with other essences such as Pine, Rock Water, or Walnut.

Best supportive technique
Read "Healing the Shame that Binds You" by John Bradshaw.
(See pp. 140–141.)

AFFIRMATION
Love from a greater source will restore me to wholeness.

Key words
POSITIVE: *Cleansing, inner purity, spiritual evolution.*
NEGATIVE: *Unclean, impure, physical obsessiveness.*

Challenge
To go beyond desiring bodily health and to seek the true healing of spiritual evolution.

CASE STUDY

Hannah, age 32, was a yoga teacher.
She developed a severe rash all around her throat and chest. She had tried fasting, homeopathy, and herbal medicine. She was highly critical of herself because she felt that as a yoga teacher her body should be immaculate. The more she did to get rid of the rash, the worse it got. Hannah took Crab Apple in a dosage bottle, as compresses on her throat, and added to a bath. Within a week the rash had disappeared.

Hannah then began to talk to friends about her experience with her own yoga teacher, whom she had traveled to see six months previously. He had been very critical of her, and she realized that she had taken his criticism very seriously and felt so ashamed that it was even too painful to think about her humiliating experience. Hannah was then ready to move on to Rock Water and other remedies and slowly she began to heal emotionally.

FOLKLORE AND USAGE

❁ The apple has powerful associations with the Fall of Mankind. Deep mysteries are contained within this myth. One way in which we can understand its meaning is to learn that, through choosing to accept the gifts of the five senses, we have to accept the inevitable bitterness of being cast out of Paradise. We lose the innocence of being pure spirit and come to terms with the imperfections of the physical plane. This was Eve's gift to Adam in the Garden of Eden, and as such contains not just the "curse" but the blessing and the secret of how to return. We may have lost our innocence in choosing to eat the fruit, but we have also lost our ignorance. So the secret we learn is that only by losing our innocence, grieving over its loss, and becoming ready to be in control of our senses, do we find a way to the ecstatic consciousness of Paradise regained. Thus the bitter taste of separation from the Source becomes the impetus for renewing wholeness. Within the crabbed and ancient lies the purity of lost innocence.

❁ The fruit contains minerals that cleanse the system. Its sharp astringent taste curtails the appetite.

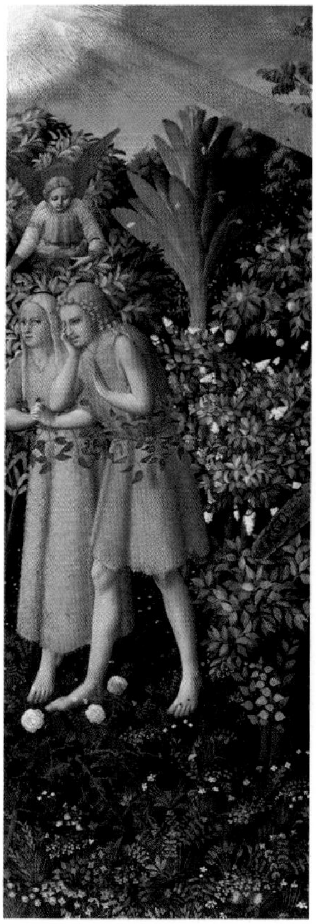

LEFT *The apple symbolizes temptation in the Bible, as the gift from Eve to Adam that led to their expulsion from the Garden of Eden.*

Oenothera hookeri
Evening Primrose

EVENING PRIMROSE *isn't a primrose at all. It belongs to the willowherb family, which grows throughout the world, mostly in temperate regions. There are 100 species of the Evening Primrose, which is native to North and South America. It grows from Kansas to Nevada and even flourishes in the desert as far as Northern Mexico. An additional number of species have hybridized in Europe where they grow wild in disturbed ground.*

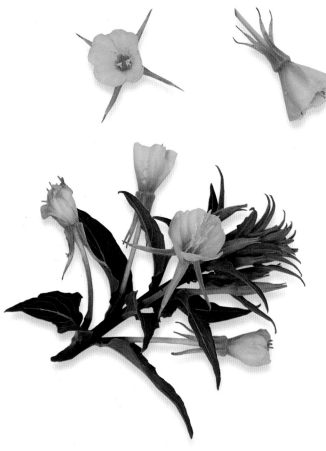

ABOVE *Each flower has four reflexed sepals, four petals, prominent stamens, and a cross shaped stigma.*

SIGNATURE

❧ *The moon replenishes missing feminine strength* ❧

Name
It is also called yellow evening primrose or sundrops. *Oenothera* **comes from the Greek** *oinos,* **meaning wine, and** *thera* **from** *therapea,* **to heal.** *Hookeri* **comes from Hooker, the English botanist who actually discovered the plant.**

Color/shape
It is a biennial, with a rosette of lance-shaped leaves in the first year and a leafy flowering spike up to 5ft. (1.5m) tall in the second. The scented, showy yellow flowers open in the evening.

Habitat and growth pattern
The evening primrose flowers open wide at dusk and release their scent to attract moths. It is extraordinary to watch the furled petals unroll in response to the moonlight. The calyx gradually relaxes, releasing pressure until the four heart-shaped yellow petals spring free from their "womb" and fully expand.

    In its first year, the evening primrose puts out only clusters of leaves. During its second year, the plants send up tall flowering stalks. The cup-shaped flowers are initially pale yellow, becoming orange-red, as if nourished and warmed by their magnetic connection to the moon. Orange is the color of the energy of reproduction.

FOLKLORE AND USAGE

❀ In some theories of the origins of our planetary system, it was the moon who gave birth to the earth, not the other way around. So this plant that is attracted to the moon is turning back to its original source for nourishment – ancestral Mother Moon.

❀ Evening primrose oil is derived from a very close relative of this plant, *Oenothera biennis.* It has proved a valuable remedy because it contains nutrients that help with menstruation and prepare the body for pregnancy. It is also used to treat a number of other complaints including eczema, asthma, and acne. It is sometimes referred to as "mother's milk for adults."

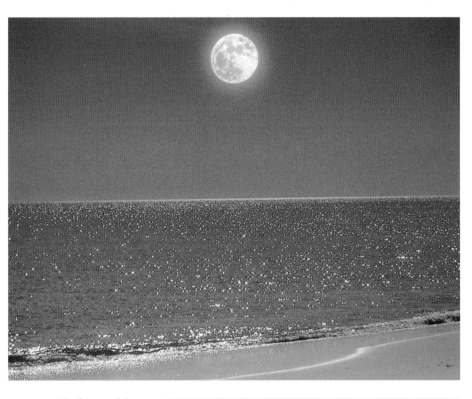

Key words

POSITIVE: *Opening to emotional nourishment, open to healing emotional pain, warmth toward others.*
NEGATIVE: *Rejection, fear of parenthood, sense of deprivation.*

Challenge

To discern what love and warmth is available in your environment and to stay connected to it.

NOTES

Therapeutic actions
Heals painful early emotions absorbed from the mother; develops the ability to open up emotionally and form deep, committed relationships.

Method of making essence
Sun method, with moon exposure.

Ways of using and use in combination
Use with Chicory or Self-heal.

Best supportive technique
Psychotherapy.

ABOVE *The flowers of the evening primrose open at dusk and should be collected for use in the moonlight.*

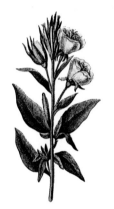

OENOTHERA HOOKERI

CASE STUDY

Karen was extremely unhappy with her work and her college life. She had experienced utmost difficulty in relating to other women, feeling rejected and humiliated in a series of jobs and college courses.
She was having great difficulty in knowing what to do with her life; whatever she started seemed to collapse because of her unbearable sensitivity. As she worked with her flower essence therapist, she realized to her dismay that she was often critical and aloof.

After taking Evening Primrose for a couple of weeks, Karen began to realize the depth of her alienation from her mother. Slowly it dawned on her, with the help of her therapist, that her mother had tried to abort her. This explained a lot to her about her aversion to many women and why she definitely did not want children, although she was happily married.

Karen began to train as an osteopath and became friends with her fellow students. She passed her exams with honors.

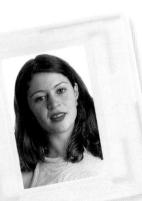

LEFT *Karen had always had a poor relationship with her mother, but Evening Primrose helped her to overcome her feelings of being unwanted.*

Olea europoea

Olive

THE OLEACEAE *family likes the dry, rocky places of the Mediterranean, Africa to Central Asia, and Australasia. It contains a wide variety of important economic and horticulturally valuable plants –* Fraxinus *(ash),* Syringa *(lilac), and* Olea *(olive).* Olea europoea *is native to the hot Mediterranean countries but also loves California. Grown in huge groves, it is very important economically for its abundant and nutritious oil. Its wood is hard and smooth-grained – ideal for carving.*

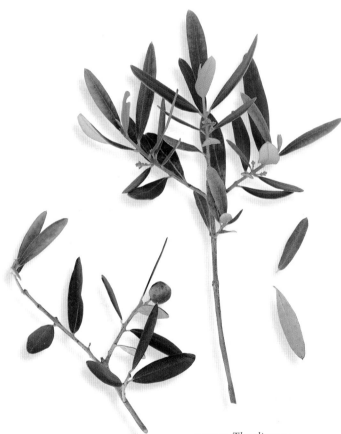

ABOVE *The olive tree has silvery-green foliage. It is a fruitful tree and may live up to 1,500 years.*

SIGNATURE

Hold the power of the sun to renew and restore

Name
Olea europoea, **European olive. One of the oldest European trees.**

Color/shape
Clusters of tiny white four-petaled flowers appear in midsummer, followed by red or purple oval fruits – the edible olive. White represents transcendent energy and four is grounding.

Habitat and growth pattern
Olive trees can live to 1,500 years or more, giving abundantly of their fruits until the last. They develop slowly taking ten years to grow to their full height of 16ft. (5m) tall. As they age they become extremely gnarled. In contrast, their simple silvery foliage stays clear and light. Olive branches bend low giving way to the forces of gravity gracefully. They bend with the aging forces that allow them to regenerate simply and easily.

When cut down they then renew themselves again by sprouting new growth. They love the sun and will not fruit unless they have plenty of warmth. This suggests that, using solar power, they give of themselves enormously using minimum effort.

FOLKLORE AND USAGE

❋ Archeology shows that the olive has played a large part in the culture of early European civilizations, serving as a symbol of immortality and fruitfulness. In Greek myth, Athens was named after the goddess Athena because she created the most acceptable gift for humankind – the olive tree. Apollo, the sun god, was also connected to the olive tree.

❋ In the Old Testament it was the olive branch that the dove brought to show Noah that the flood was over and peace had returned to the earth. In Judaism, it is considered sacred and used for fueling the Sabbath lamp.

❋ Jesus went to the Mount of Olives to rest before he was arrested and taken for trial.

❋ Two olive branches encircle the world as a symbol of peace on the flag of the United Nations.

❋ Olive oil, which has extremely nutritious and health-giving properties, has been used for healing internally and externally for thousands of years.

Key words

POSITIVE: *Renewed by
spiritual source, perseverance,
understanding correct
energy use.*
NEGATIVE: *Exhaustion,
depletion, unwise
use of energy.*

Challenge

*To attune to forces beyond
the physical in anticipation
of renewal.*

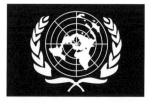

NOTES

Therapeutic actions
*Restoration after "burn
out" of any sort, including
long illness or prolonged
emotional stress such as
divorce. Olive helps to
understand and correct the
misuse of energy and
enables understanding and
contact with the spiritual
sources of renewal.*

Method of
making essence
*Sun method. Pick a leaf to
cover your hand and place
the blooms upon it before
putting them quickly
in the water.*

Ways of using and
use in combination
*Dosage bottle, baths,
and ointments.*

Best supportive technique
*Take some time every day
to have meditative rest in
contact with the earth and
sun when possible. If this
is not possible, use sitting
yoga postures.*

LEFT *Symbolizing peace,
two olive branches are
portrayed on the
United Nations' flag.*

BELOW *The dove brought
back an olive branch to the
ark to prove to Noah that
the Flood had receded.*

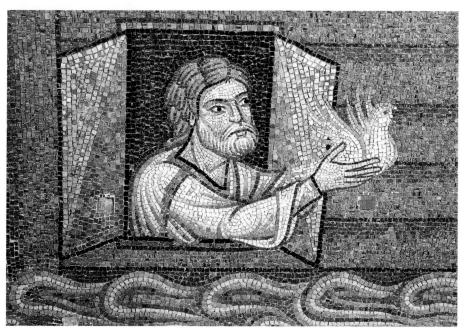

**Claire worked hard
all day, shopped in her
lunch break, then came
home to look after
her children.**
After she had put them
to bed, she watched TV
until she went to sleep.
She began to get
frequent colds and feel
run down and
exhausted but didn't
understand why
because she had a good
diet and slept for seven
hours a night. After
taking Olive for a week
Claire realized that she
never really rested. She
saw that time in front of
the television was
actually keeping her
mind spinning all the
time and giving her
frantic dreams. She
began to slow herself
down during the day by
eating quietly in the
office and turning the
television off at
9:00 p.m., to give
herself a quiet hour
before going to sleep at
night. After another
month of Olive essence
she decided to work
parttime so that she
would have more of the
"quiet time" for herself
that she was beginning
to truly cherish. She
stopped getting colds
and felt refreshed and
truly revitalized.

Ornithogalum umbellatum

Star of Bethlehem

S TAR OF BETHLEHEM *belongs to the Hyacinth branch of the* Liliaceae *or Onion family, which is one of the largest families of flowering plants. It is of outstanding beauty and many of its members have uses as essences. It is a cosmopolitan perennial but grows widely in Europe, Turkey, Syria, Lebanon, Israel, and North Africa. Botanists don't know whether it is native to Britain or not but it grows in profusion in East Anglia.*

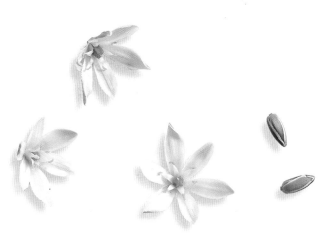

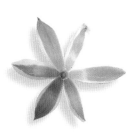

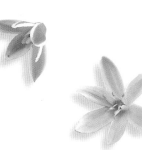

ABOVE *The Star of Bethlehem has a six-pointed star shaped pure white flower.*

SIGNATURE

The perfect symmetry of heaven and earth soothes discord past and present

Name
Its name is Star of Bethlehem, not only because it is connected to the star of Christ's Nativity but also because it grows in profusion in Palestine. It is called "dove's dung" by the Arabs. *Umbellatum* **relates to its umbel shape;** *umbellis* **is Latin for parasol. It is called nap-at-noon in the United States.**

Color/shape
Three sepals and three petals identical in shape make up the interlacing triangles of the Star of Bethlehem, symbolizing energy moving from the heaven downward and the earth upward to make perfect harmony. Each petal is backed with a broad green strip and the long thin leaves are mid-green with a central silvery-white stripe.

Green is the color of balance and the reverse patterning of flower and leaf is another sign of the balancing of opposites. In the center of the flower is a six-pointed crown of stamens tipped with golden yellow stigmas. The crown was a symbol of the heavenly order of thought worthy of a king.

Habitat and growth pattern
Because of the watery round nature of the bulb, the lily family is associated with the soothing properties of the moon. A fibrous sheath covers the bulb and the flowers are ultrasensitive to light so they open fully only in the sunshine. This symbolizes our sensitivity to shock and shows us how to protect ourselves.

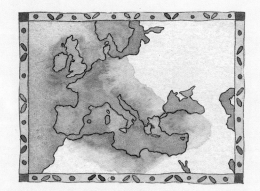

ABOVE *Europe and The Mediterranean is the natural home of the Star of Bethlehem.*

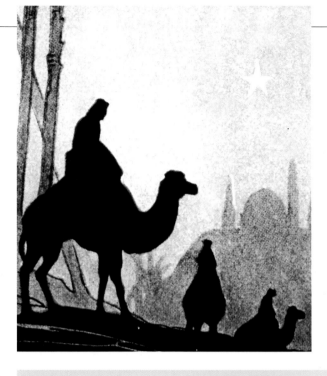

AFFIRMATION
From the stability of peace I gently release past shocks.

FOLKLORE AND USAGE

❁ Muslim pilgrims were said to have dried Star of Bethlehem bulbs to eat on their way to Mecca.

❁ Homeopaths have been known to make a tincture and use it to treat some cases of cancer.

Key words
POSITIVE: *Unnumbing, peace, tranquillity, soothing.*
NEGATIVE: *Shock, trauma, numbing from past trauma and shock.*

Challenge
To find rest and recuperation through experiencing the harmony of heaven on earth.

LEFT *Native to Israel and Palestine, the Star of Bethlehem plant is also closely associated with Christ's Nativity star.*

NOTES

Therapeutic actions
Releases the deadening effect of unresolved shock and trauma and helps to restore mental, emotional, and physical equilibrium.

Method of making essence
Boiling method. Pick them when they are fully open with a small piece of the main stem.

Ways of using and use in combination
A main ingredient of Rescue Remedy or Five Flower Formula. Especially effective as baths, but also as dosage and creams.

Best supportive technique
Take time out to take care of yourself.

CASE STUDY

Nadine was normally a happy balanced person but lately had been feeling depressed and anxious and couldn't figure out what was wrong.
During flower essence counseling she realized that she was brooding on the messy end of a relationship a few years back and other events were troubling her that she thought she had resolved. She began to understand that she hadn't felt right since she was involved in a car accident a couple of months before. Because no one was hurt she discounted the shock of being close to danger.

After bathing and dosing herself with Star of Bethlehem for a week Nadine felt soothed. She saw that the accident was

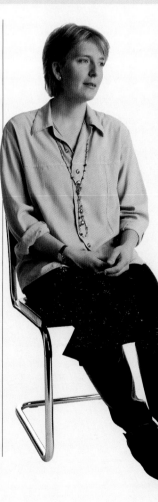

necessary to make her more alive to past emotional shocks she had numbed herself against. With the sense of security that Star of Bethlehem gave her she was able to take action to complete much unfinished business.

LEFT *Nadine found that Star of Bethlehem essence helped her to confront past traumas and shock.*

Paphiopedilum insigne

Himalayan Slipper Orchid

AFFIRMATION
I am rooted in the
divine order.

Key words
POSITIVE: *Self-exploration.*
NEGATIVE: *Ignorance of self.*

Challenge
Know thyself.

T HE PAPHIOPEDILUM *or slipper orchids are native to southern Asia and grow from the Himalayas eastward to New Guinea. They are a genus of about 60 species of evergreen orchids, mainly terrestrial (growing on the ground). Some of them are epiphytic, that is to say they grow upon other plants, mainly trees, living on moisture from the atmosphere and humus from crevices in bark. Others are lithophytic, growing on rocks or among stones. They grow from sea level to more than 6,500ft. (2,000m).*

SIGNATURE

All knowledge lies within

Name
Paphiopedilum means
a pouch on a stalk, and
insigne means
remarkable.

Color/shape
Himalayan slipper orchid
flowers are very glossy.
They usually grow alone
but they sometimes pair
up on stems that can grow
to 1ft. (30cm) tall. They
are 4–5in. (10–13cm)
across. The usual color is
green with white waves at
the tip but they can be
spotted and streaked
with brown. The wings
are usually yellow-green
with bronze veins but
the amount of shading
and spotting varies
considerably from
flower to flower.

The most important
feature of Himalayan
slipper orchid is the shape
of the deep, central flower
petal in the form of a
pouch that looks like a
wooden clog. The depth
of this central flower petal

symbolizes the depth to
which this essence allows
us to enter into ourselves.
Shoes can symbolize
many things but here the
symbolism relates to how
we understand our path
in life, so that we can
walk it with awareness.

Habitat and
growth pattern
The Himalayas have
always been known, in
the East, for their great
spiritual importance as
a sanctuary for men and
women seeking a pure
atmosphere for inner
contemplation.

The Himalayan slipper
orchid doesn't create
pseudo–bulbs (swollen
segments), unlike many
other orchids, so it
signifies simplicity and
being true to ourselves.
These are terrestrial
orchids, indicating that
we need to get to know
ourselves while we are
on earth, not wait until
we die for a miracle!

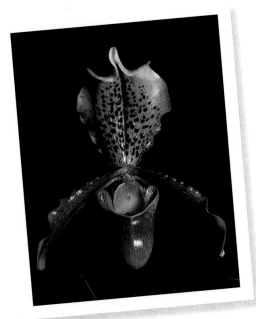

ABOVE *The central flower petal of the Himalayan slipper orchid is in the form of a deep pouch.*

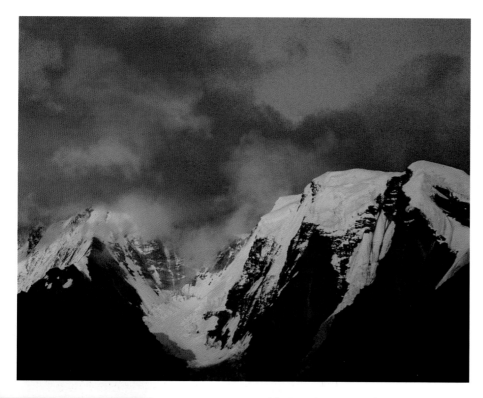

ABOVE *The Himalayan mountains invite contemplation and spirituality as does the Himalayan slipper orchid, a native of this majestic mountain range.*

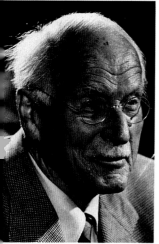

ABOVE *Psychotherapist Carl Jung (1875–1962). Psychotherapy is a supportive technique to flower essence therapy.*

RIGHT *Crystals, such as amethyst, can be worn as a support to flower essence therapy.*

NOTES

Therapeutic actions
For knowledge of life, to discover the reason for our existence; supports us in finding ourselves through helping us to access our subconscious; helps us to recognize and accept ourselves; enhances every type of counseling or psychotherapy work.

Method of making essence
Crystal method. Read Andreas Korte's book (see Bibliography pp. 140–141).

Ways of using and use in combination
Use alone, after working with emotional and mental blocks.

Best supportive technique
Deep inside ourselves, some time sooner or later, we have to find the answers to these questions: Who am I really? What is my task? What am I doing here? Write your responses spontaneously. Also psychotherapy; wearing amethyst gems.

Geoffrey, a 59-year-old man, worked as an advertising executive. He had suffered a series of illnesses culminating in a serious bout of bronchitis that lasted for six months. He ate well, exercised regularly, had a good marriage but was still depressed. His homeopath suggested that he should have some counseling but he told her that "he was not interested in himself." After taking Himalayan Slipper Orchid, Geoffrey began to have vivid dreams, including one about a fox who lived in his attic. He realized that the fox was his secret self. He began to write down his dreams and became very excited about the richness of his inner life and how full of meaning it was. He realized that he had been so focused on earning a living and having the things that he thought brought happiness, that he had neglected his reason for living, his humanity.

Three weeks later, he completely recovered from bronchitis. He continued his journal, he felt much more excited about life and became much happier and contented.

Prunella vulgaris

Self-heal

THE APOTHECARY *shops of the Middle Ages were full of medicines for infusions, tinctures, and ointments made from the* Labiatae *(mint) family. Other members of the mint family tend to have smaller flowers and frequently contain healing oils. Self-heal relates more to the mental aspect of healing than the physical. It is widespread in Europe, Asia, North Africa, Australia, and North America.*

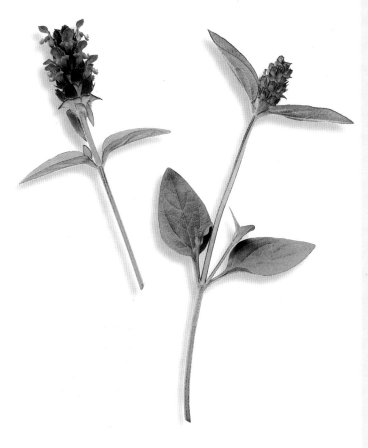

ABOVE *Violet flowers grow in tight minaretlike spikes from midsummer. The leaves of the plant are shiny green.*

❧ *The power to heal ourselves lies within* ❧

Name

The name self-heal is self-explanatory. Self-heal is also known in England as hook-heal, sickly-wort, and carpenter's herb. The upper lip of the self-heal flower is clearly in the shape of a hook. Bill hooks and sickles were the main causes of wounds in the medieval farming community. In Germany it is called *Brunella* because it was used to treat *die Breuen*, or sore throat. The small flowers look like a throat that has swollen glands.

Color/shape

Self-heal flowers are a radiant violet-blue color. Each small flower is two-lipped, with a hood-shaped upper lip and a spreading lower lip to guide bees to the pollen. This makes it look like a protective cave.

As many as 12 of these small flowers climb upward on one stem, little minarets of exotic color among the cool green leaves. The blue color nourishes and soothes the

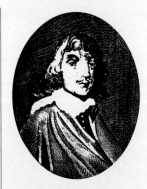

ABOVE *Nicholas Culpeper (1616–54), the English herbalist, held self-heal in high regard.*

throat chakra, and the violet color relates to the crown chakra and the power of the creative imagination to transform.

Habitat and growth pattern

Self-heal grows prolifically in grassland, waste ground, lawns, and open spaces in woods.

The fruit is composed of four nutlets. As the number four is concerned with being grounded, so self-heal helps to generate creative soothing thoughts that become grounded in the body.

FOLKLORE AND USAGE

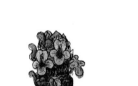

AFFIRMATION
I awaken the self-healing
power within me.

Key words
POSITIVE: *Motivation and
direction from within.*
NEGATIVE: *Powerlessness
about healing.*

Challenge
*To be in touch with the
healer within.*

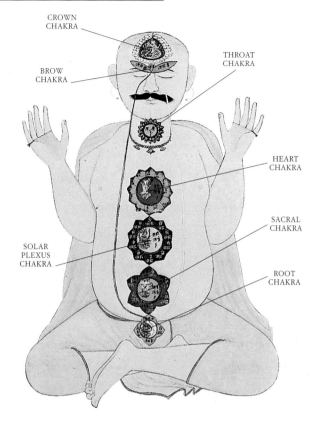

ABOVE *The self-heal flowers
are violet-blue, colors that nourish
the throat and crown chakras.*

PRUNELLA VULGARIS

❋ Culpeper says that self-heal is "a special remedy for inward and outward wounds, made into a syrup for internal injuries and for outward wounds as unguents and plasters."

❋ *Prunella vulgaris* was cited in Chinese medical literature during the Han dynasty, 206 B.C.E. – 220 C.E., to balance and harmonize disturbed liver energy. The flowers are still used in Chinese medicine as healing for disturbed liver energy in children. Making sure the liver is functioning well is an important first step for the Western naturopath.

❋ Self-heal is used in Western medicine as a spring tonic, as a general tonic in convalescence, or as a gargle for sore throats. On a mental level too, it helps us to take the first steps toward healing ourself.

NOTES

Therapeutic actions
Helps us when we don't know where to turn for healing; motivates us to be well and to find a way through; helps to clarify what we need to do; encourages us to persevere with any healing plan.

**Method of
making essence**
Sun method.

**Ways of using and
use in combination**
In a dosage bottle added to any other combination where self-healing needs to be activated, whether emotional, mental, or physical (for example, use it with Star of Bethlehem for shock or with Crab Apple for skin problems); use as fresh plant tincture, a flower essence, and as a base for blends of flower essences and aromatherapy oils.

Best supportive technique
Self-heal itself is the best support for any technique of healing. Use it for whatever level of healing you need to address.

CASE STUDY

**Kenneth, a 35-year-old,
had lung cancer.**
He was terrified of a recurrence of his illness. After taking Self-heal, he decided to try acupuncture, which worked well for him. Two years later, he reported that he was "fit as a fiddle," and that the essence had helped him find the way to prevent the cancer reoccuring.

Prunus cerasifera
Cherry Plum

CHERRY *Plum belongs to the large and important* Rosaceae *or Rose family. The fossil record shows this family to be among the most ancient. It includes apples, cherries, plums, peaches, raspberries, and strawberries as well as a multitude of flowering ornamental roses. Cherry plum is native to the Balkans and south-east Europe and was brought to Britain where it has naturalized, often in hedges.*

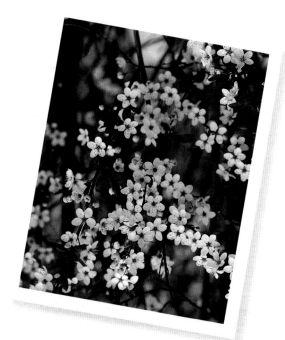

ABOVE *The cherry plum tree is often grown just for its early, magnificent blossom that appears in February.*

SIGNATURE

❦ *Courage to face darkness, brings hope of light* ❦

Name
Cherry plum is also called *Myrobalan*. **Prunus – a plum tree,** *cerasifera* **– means bearing cherries or cherry-like fruits.**

Color/shape
The cherry plum flowers are bowl-shaped 1in. (2.5cm) across and are borne along bare shoots in the early spring before the dark green leaves appear. It has the earliest flowering of its species, braving the world before the winter ends in February. The flowers blooming with white intensity against the brownish-black bark while the darkness of winter is all around suggest a willingness to brave the most difficult times and bring light to dark places.

The flowers are pure white with five petals and five sepals with numerous stamens. They often bloom singly, sometimes in clusters. Five is the number of the senses and pure white represents purity – so cherry plum brings purity and light back to our sensory experience.

Habitat and
growth pattern
It is a deciduous tree or shrub that grows up to 10–12ft. (3–4m) high. The young twigs are sometimes thorny.

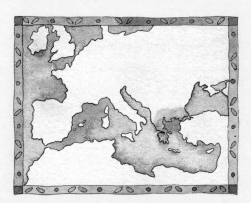

ABOVE *Cherry plum originally came from the Balkans and South-eastern Europe.*

AFFIRMATION
I face my inner darkness protected by a benevolent higher power.

Key words
POSITIVE: *Self-control, trust in a higher power.*
NEGATIVE: *Fear of losing control of self, of breaking down, giving way to harmful impulses.*

Challenge
To surrender to a higher power that can nourish the personality with courage and peace.

FOLKLORE AND USAGE

❁ Cherry plum is often planted for hedging and shelter belts around orchards, suggesting its protective quality. Also used as stock for grafting selected varieties of plums and gages because of its strength. The fruit is small and cherrylike, ripening from a pale glossy green to red or yellow and can be eaten in warm climates where it becomes fully ripe.

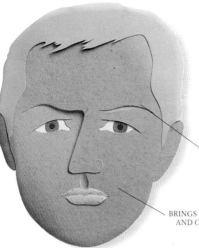

LEFT *Cherry Plum essence helps the mind to surrender to a higher power, bringing peace and calm.*

HELPS WITH SELF-CONTROL

BRINGS PEACE AND CALM

NOTES

Therapeutic actions
Releases the mind from tormenting thoughts of harming self or another, of going mad. Brings peace and calm. Gives mental strength.

Method of making essence
Boiling method. Use the flowering twigs with the flowers from as many bushes as possible.

Ways of using and use in combination
Dosage bottle, baths, creams, but most important, it is one of the major ingredients in Rescue Remedy or Five Flower Remedy.

Best supportive technique
To practice centering within and invoking your higher power for support and guidance.

CASE STUDY

Katherine had suffered physical abuse as a child that had left her emotionally scarred. Flower essences and counseling over a number of years had given her the support she needed and she had become generally happy with her life. She was therefore very shocked when she was taking care of a four–year–old girl for a friend that she was tormented by the thought of smacking her. She knew that this was not in her nature but she was terrified of losing control. Taking Cherry Plum for only two days eliminated these thoughts completely, and she was able to look after her friend's child in peace.

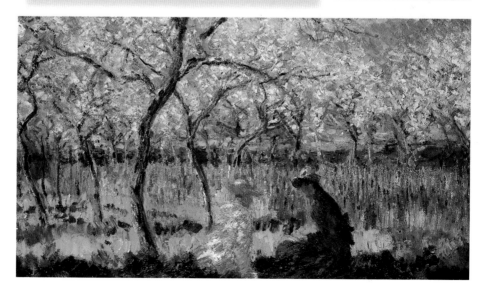

RIGHT *Cherry plum trees are traditionally planted as hedging around orchards to give shelter to fruiting trees.*

Quercus robur

Oak

Oak *belongs to the Fagaceae family, which also contains the beeches and the sweet chestnuts. There are 450 species of oaks in the world ranging from trees to bush and scrub, both evergreen and deciduous. Oak is widespread and will often dominate woods. This is the English oak often called* Quercus pedunculata.

BELOW *The leaves and flowers appear in May. Male flowers hang in loose clusters of catkins.*

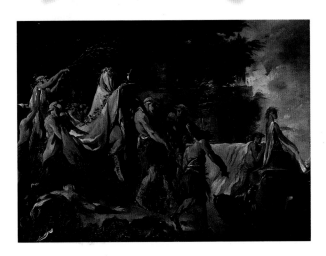

LEFT *The Druids use the oak tree in their magical rites and rituals.*

Deep roots ensure endurance in selfless support of others

Name
Quercus **is Latin for oak, *robur* means sturdy strength.**

Color/shape
Male and female flowers both grow on the same tree at midsummer at the turning of the year. The yellowish male catkins droop in loose clusters. The less conspicuous and fewer yellowish-green female flowers make a globe from overlapping scales that will harden to form the cup for the acorn. This female flower is the powerhouse of future oaks.

"Mighty oaks from tiny acorns grow."

Habitat and growth pattern
Oak trees live to a great age, maturing slowly, taking 60 years to produce their first full crop of catkins. They may live on for around 800 years. They grow to 110ft. (30m) high with girths of 30–40ft. (9–12m). The roots are reputed to reflect this size deep underground.

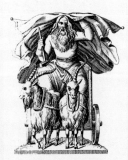

ABOVE *The acorn is sacred to Thor, the Scandinavian thunder god.*

They are sturdy and their trunks are extremely gnarled. The heavy horizontal branches look like arms outstretched, defying gravity, ready to help all who go by. The oak's reputation as serving others with great devotion is reinforced by the fact that each tree can support up to 43 species of varied flora and fauna. Oak can be hollowed out to a shell by wood-burrowing insects and still stand for generations before suddenly crumbling. This can happen to a person who needs oak; they soldier on helping others till they completely collapse.

FOLKLORE AND USAGE

AFFIRMATION
Rooted in nature,
I use my strength
flexibly and wisely.

Key words
POSITIVE: *Flexible
strength, surrender, takes
support for self.*
NEGATIVE: *Depression from
long struggle, overresponsible
for others, chronic
exhaustion.*

Challenge
*To let go of struggle and
persevere with flexibility
and support.*

❊ Acorns (from *korn,* which means oak seed in Danish) are said to have been the first food in many cultures. In herbalism, oak bark has been used throughout the ages for its strong toning effect on the mucous membranes throughout the body, treating gastroenteritis and severe diarrhea, fevers, and sore throats. Externally it is used on varicose veins, hemorrhoids, chilblains, frostbite, sweaty feet, burns, and skin diseases.

❊ The lumber is hard and tough and used in the construction of ships and the frames of houses.

❊ In Western cultures it is sacred to the earth mother, Juno, Jupiter, and the Scandinavian god Thor. In most European countries it symbolizes heroism. According to mythology, oak was the first tree and the Romans believed that it gave birth to humankind. The oak is used magically at all the major Druidic festivals. In Christianity it is a symbol of Christ's steadfastness, and for the Jewish people it is a symbol of divine presence. In China it symbolizes rigid strength because it does not bend with the wind and so can break.

BELOW *The horizontal branches of the oak give it great breadth and stature, just like the people who may need the essence.*

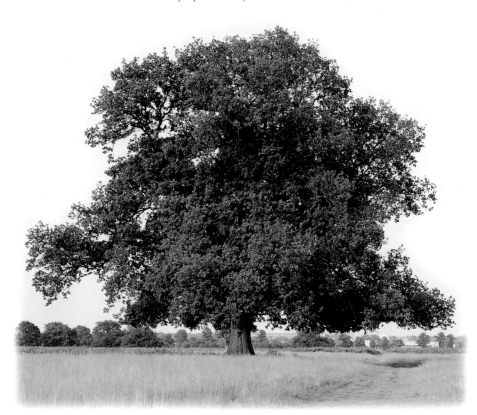

NOTES

Therapeutic actions
Helps to release struggle; encourages us to shed the burdens of others; restores fortitude; brings strength with flexibility.

Method of making essence
Sun method. Gather the female catkins only from a grove of oaks using many different trees.

Ways of using and use in combination
Dosage, baths, and as a lotion, particularly on shoulders and neck.

Best supportive technique
Take frequent breaks to do something just for fun; delegate.

CASE STUDY

Felicity was recovering from cancer and following a strict diet. She found cooking for her new diet very wearing. After taking Oak, Felicity decided to join a cancer support group and attend Ayurvedic cooking classes so that she could continue on her diet more inventively. She felt renewed strength and vitality return.

Rosa canina

Wild Rose

THE ROSE *family* Rosaceae *is a large family of woody and herbaceous plants that are distributed worldwide, mostly in temperate areas. The family includes apples, pears, cherries, and plums. The remains of wild rosehips have been found at prehistoric dwelling sites, which suggests that roses have been grown for thousands of years.*

Certainly the beauty of their blooms and perfumes has inspired mystics and poets from time immemorial. This wild rose is the ancestor of many beautiful cultivated roses. It brightens hedgerows and scrubland throughout Britain.

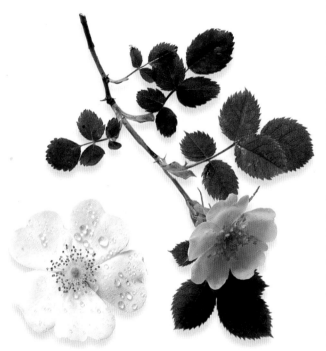

ABOVE *The wild rose is a vigorous and thorny climber that grows on waste ground and in hedgerows.*

SIGNATURE

❦ *Celebrating life as a mixture of pleasure and pain* ❧

Name
The wild rose is known as the dog rose or *Rosa canina* because the thorns look like dogs' teeth and because it is supposed to be able to cure the bite of a mad dog.

Color/shape
Rosa canina **is a deciduous shrub with arched, downward-curving branches with thorns. The rose flowers have five large flat heart-shaped petals that are white, sometimes tinged with pink, or deep pink all over. The soft petals and the sensuous smell invite us into physicality but the sharp thorns warn us that life is also painful.**

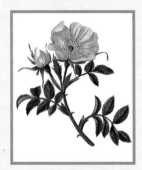

ROSA CANINA

Habitat and growth pattern
The wild rose grows on the fringes of woods in hedgerows and on stony slopes. It pulls itself toward the light through hedges and vegetation by means of its stout hooked thorns, which are also used for defense. Similarly, what can hurt us can also, used rightly, provide strong support.

FOLKLORE AND USAGE

✿ The rose has always been associated with love. It also reminds us of the transitory nature of life on earth; in love we have to face and accept the pain of separation from the loved one.

✿ In Hindu ceremonies a water sprinkler shaped like a flower is filled with rose water and is sprinkled on shrines for symbolic purification.

✿ The fruit of the rose, the rose hip, is like a bright red flask, fleshy and rich in vitamin C. Vitamin C helps prevent disease and must have sustained our ancestors throughout many hard winters. It is hard to obtain the goodness from the hips. It is easy to choke on even the slightest remains of hairs from inside the fruit unless the boiled juice is thoroughly strained before drinking.

AFFIRMATION
I grasp life fully,
willingly facing
pleasure and pain.

Key words
POSITIVE: *Enthusiasm,
vitality, purpose.*
NEGATIVE: *Resignation,
apathy, avoidance,
acceptance.*

Challenge
*To be willing to face your
pain in order to move
through it. To be ready then
to create a life about which
you can be enthusiastic.*

CASE STUDY

**John had been
diagnosed as diabetic
for over a year.**
He had cut down on his
social life because it was
too much bother to
organize his food if he
went out. As he
experienced slight side-
effects from his diabetic
drugs he stopped taking
them. He decided to see
a flower essence
therapist on the advice
of a friend.

After taking Wild
Rose for two weeks,
John realized that he
had been neglecting his
health and well-being
and decided to try
another sort of diabetic
drug. He also began to
talk to his friends about
his dietary needs. After
taking Wild Rose for
another month, he
realized that the
sweetness had gone out
of his life after the
sudden death of his
meditation teacher, his
guide and close friend.
A month later, after
some counseling, John
began to grieve more
openly for his teacher,
sharing his deep
experience of loss with
fellow students and
friends. Gradually he
regained his interest in
life, deciding to plant a
memorial garden for his
teacher. Through
tending the garden
(a rose garden) he felt
more alive.

NOTES

Therapeutic actions
*Supports a renewed
interest in life and health,
and should be borne in
mind for those who have
degenerative diseases;
reminds those who are,
due to prolonged apathy,
disconnected from their life
that it is full of beauty as
well as pain, and that there
is a meaning and power in
being in a physical world.*

**Method of
making essence**
*Boiling method. Collect
blooms with a short length
of stalk and some leaves
from different bushes.*

**Ways of using and use
in combination**
*Dosage bottle; make into a
lotion and rub all around
the heart; use with Self-heal,
Zinnia, Crowea, Thyme, or
Borage, whichever are most
appropriate to your needs.*

Best supportive technique
*Ask yourself the following
questions: When did I lose
interest in life? What
would make me want to
live again?*

*What's stopping me?
What is my next step?
Read love poetry and
write a poem about your
feelings; smell the flowers;
grow flowers; aromatherapy,
especially using rose and
pine oil to invigorate the
physical body; use a
selection of flower
essences in the
bathtub with or
in a diffuser.*

ABOVE *As well as taking
Wild Rose essence, read
poetry to remind yourself that
life is full of love and beauty.*

BELOW *Aromatherapy
massage with rose and pine
oils will support the use of
Wild Rose essence.*

PINE OIL

Solanum quadriloculatum

Wild Potato Bush

THE WILD POTATO *belongs to the* Solanaceae *family, which includes potatoes, tomatoes, eggplants, S. melongena, green and red peppers. The great concentration of this family in South America has led many to believe that it may have originated there. The* Solanaceae *are found throughout most tropical and temperate regions. Many beautiful* Solanaceae *are now cultivated as ornamentals in Europe, such as the Chilean potato tree, the potato vine, and the Christmas cherry from South America, and the kangaroo apple from Australia.* Solanum quadriloculatum *is found in various habitats in central Australia where it can be frequently seen along roadsides.*

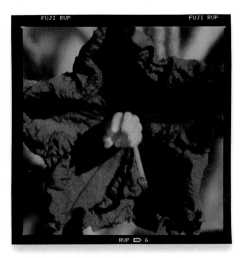

ABOVE *The wild potato bush has purple five-petaled flowers that have a bright yellow center.*

SIGNATURE

❦ *Remain unhindered by the body's limitations* ❧

Name

The word *Solanum* goes back to ancient times, coming from *sol*, meaning the sun. It is also the name of the nightshade plants, so there is a strong association with the relationship between darkness and light. Alchemists and mystics express this paradoxical quality when they talk about the body. They see us as endarkened because the vastness of spirit is trapped in the body, but equally, the human body is the life form in which we can realize the light. So there is a magical otherworldly quality to the name of this plant.

Color/shape

Wild potato bush has five-pointed purplish-blue flowers. This deep purple color is connected to the vibrational energy of the third eye. Since the five points of the flower relate to the five senses (seeing, hearing, tasting, smelling, touching), the flower suggests that we can have dominion over the senses. Each five-sided flower has vibrant yellow clustered stamens in its center that point strongly upward. Yellow suggests fiery strength, so the plant is concerned with giving strength and energizing the body by controlling it.

Habitat and growth pattern

The tomatolike fruits of the wild potato will cause severe discomfort if you eat them, but many native *Solanum* species are edible. Many of these plants are both poisonous and medicinal, such as deadly nightshade, jimson weed, or stramonium, which in small doses can be used to make powerful homeopathic medicines.

The fact that there are so many foods in this family implies a strong relationship to the physical body. There is also a close connection with the mind, because in this family there are psychotropic plants that can have a powerful effect on changing the nature of our consciousness. The thorn apple *Datura stramonium*, for instance, is used by Native Americans to loosen the ethereal body from the material body, within appropriate ritual, to enable them to meet with their ancestors.

So this family offers us a spectrum of possibilities: looking beautiful for us, poisoning us, feeding us and, in the case of *Solanum quadriloculatum*, freeing us from restricted body consciousness.

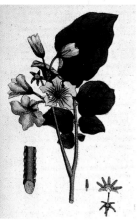

SOLANUM QUADRILOCULATUM

NOTES

Therapeutic actions
*Gives a sense of freedom
and vitality to the
physical body; especially
good during pregnancy,
and in cases of obesity,
or debilitating illness.*

**Method of
making essence**
Sun method.

**Ways of using and
use in combination**
*Take in a dosage bottle
morning and evening;
included in Dynamis
Essence (see p.125).*

**Best supportive
technique**
*Enjoyable projects that
stimulate the desire for
movement – country
walks, dance, table
tennis; use your creative
imagination if it is
difficult to get moving –
just see yourself moving
and imagine the
wonderful benefits.*

AFFIRMATION
I free myself from
all restrictions with
renewed energy.

Key words
POSITIVE: *Vitality,
freedom, transcendence.*
NEGATIVE: *Weighed down,
physically burdened,
encumbered or apathetic.*

Challenge
*To transcend limitation
through not identifying with
your physical body.*

CASE STUDY

**Marilyn had a chronic
heart condition, which
meant she had to regulate
her actions carefully, so
that exercise didn't
become stressful.**
During the summer,
Marilyn was able to warm
her body in the sun while
gardening and walking in
the countryside. During
the long winter, however,
she would lose the
impetus to move around
in any way. By the time
spring came, she would
be too scared to get
moving again. She began
to view her body as an
enemy – it was too much
trouble to care for; she'd
rather just sit and watch
the TV and vegetate.

When she took Wild
Potato Bush essence,
Marilyn sometimes felt as
if she wanted to shake.
Initially this scared her,
but as she continued she
realized that she had more
vitality in her than she had
been aware of. Her body
was telling her she was
ready to go walking again.
That spring, Marilyn lost
her apathy much more
quickly than she had in
previous years.

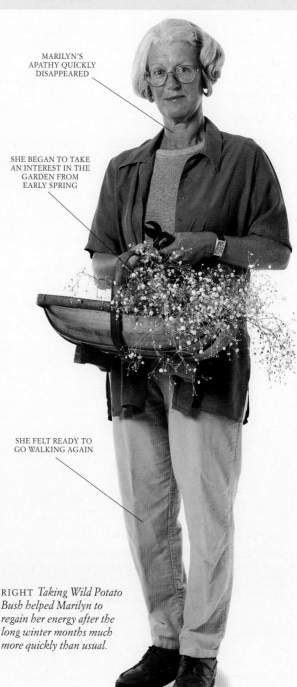

MARILYN'S
APATHY QUICKLY
DISAPPEARED

SHE BEGAN TO TAKE
AN INTEREST IN THE
GARDEN FROM
EARLY SPRING

SHE FELT READY TO
GO WALKING AGAIN

RIGHT *Taking Wild Potato
Bush helped Marilyn to
regain her energy after the
long winter months much
more quickly than usual.*

Syringa vulgaris

Lilac

SYRINGA *is a member of the* Oleacea *family of trees and shrubs that are widely distributed throughout temperate and tropical regions. The family includes olive, ash, forsythia, and jasmine.* Syringa vulgaris *is native to eastern Europe and Asia Minor where it grows to 26ft. (8m) in mountain areas. It was introduced to Britain from Persia in the 16th century. It has become naturalized in Britain and can be seen in hedgerows and thickets, and on railway embankments. It adapted incredibly well without changing its form or becoming stunted. So it helps those who need to restart their own growth with humility and flexibility. Many varieties have been cultivated from* Syringa vulgaris *and are grown as ornamentals.*

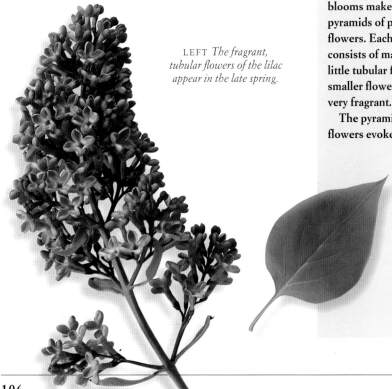

LEFT *The fragrant, tubular flowers of the lilac appear in the late spring.*

SIGNATURE

Be flexible with your feelings to bring a greater flow of energy

Name

Lilac was initially named the indigo plant in Britain. because of the blue-purple color of its flowers. It was also known as bluepipe since the hollow stems were used for pipes. *Syringa* means a tube, which relates to its therapeutic use for the spine, since the spine is essentially a tube with fine nerve fluid flowing through it.

Color/shape

Lilac is a spreading shrub that is upright when it is young. The flowers, which are 4–8in. (10–20cm) long, start to appear in the late spring. The weight of the flowers makes the branches arch elegantly. By May the blooms make large pyramids of purplish-pink flowers. Each panicle consists of many pretty little tubular four-parted smaller flowers that are very fragrant.

The pyramids of lilac flowers evoke the healing energies of the crown chakra. This shape contains the twofold meaning of integration and convergence. Once again, there is a connection with the spine. The spinal cord is where the nerves from different parts of the body converge to become integrated in the brain.

So the activities of the spine are supported from up above.

Lilac leaves make perfect heart-shapes that grow to 4in. (10cm) long. As the spine is the center of the physical body, so the heart is the center of our emotions. This suggests that lilac can support our feelings with flexibility and grace.

Habitat and growth pattern

The purple heartwood in the center of the lilac's trunk and branches suggests a healing potential that is within the spinal structure.

Key words

POSITIVE: *Flexibility,
energy-raising, releasing
past blocks.*
NEGATIVE: *Spinal rigidity,
posture, stunted character
development.*

Challenge

*To energize the spine to
allow the lifeforce to clear
blocks to development.*

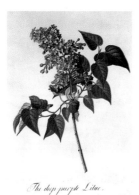

The deep purple Lilac.

SYRINGA VULGARIS

FOLKLORE AND USAGE

❀ A lilac branch was
said to signify a broken
engagement in some
19th-century English
villages.

NOTES

Therapeutic actions
*Works beneficially on all
aspects of the spine, such as
helping to calm
inflammation, trapped and
pinched nerves; acts as a
muscle relaxant, so helps to
correct posture and
increase flexibility of the
spine; activates subtle
energy channels in the
spine and balances activity
of the main spinal chakras.*

Method of making essence
Boiling method.

Ways of using and use in combination
*Use in a dosage bottle;
blend into dandelion oil,
or into a cream; use with
Dandelion, Self-heal, or
Wild Potato Bush.*

Best supportive technique
*Yoga; use with osteopathy
or cranial sacral therapy for
back problems.*

BELOW *Lilac essence is a
good remedy to take for
spinal complaints including
trapped and pinched nerves.*

HELPS INCREASE
FLEXIBILITY OF
THE SPINE

LILAC HELPS
WITH TRAPPED
OR PINCHED
NERVES

**Jenny damaged her
back in a trampoline
accident when she was
14 years old.**
She then suffered pain
from traumatized
vertebrae for 15 years.
From the age of 21, she
consulted osteopaths,
cranial osteopaths,
chiropractors, and
acupuncturists, but
although she gained
temporary relief, none
of the adjustments
would last for more
than two days.
Whenever she was
under emotional stress,
the back pain would
re-assert itself.
    Since taking Lilac,
however, Jenny has
suffered much less,
having found that the
essence lightens her
emotions and relieves
her pain.

Taraxacum officinale

Dandelion

T HE DANDELION *is a member of the Compositae family, which is the largest botanical family of plants. They grow everywhere that plant life can be supported. The hardy and vital dandelion reflects this characteristic of its family. It grows prolifically, much to the disgust of formal gardeners but to the delight of herbalists and naturalists. Compositae family members range from the common daisy to the sunflower, from the lettuce to the dahlia. Many important flower essences are made from this family. They include chicory, madia, chamomile, sunflower, and zinnia.*

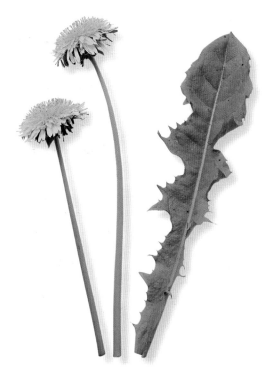

ABOVE *The dandelion has bright yellow daisylike flowers. Its spear-shaped leaves are serrated.*

SIGNATURE

Rooted yet free, energetic vitality both relaxes and invigorates a stressful life

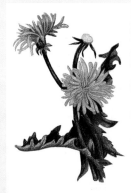

TARAXACUM OFFICINALE

Name

The word dandelion comes from the French *Dent-de-lion*, or lion's teeth, because the jagged edges of the leaves are like the teeth of a wild animal. *Taraxacum* is derived from the Greek word for edible, and *officinale* means that it is medicinal. It was also known as blow-balls and noon-head-clocks.

Color/shape

The dandelion's flower is like a fiery explosion of golden yellow. It has an outgoing character of enormous energy. Each flowerhead is made of 100 slender petals. Yet this power-packed bundle of energy is so light it only needs a slender hollow stem 3–10in. (7.5–25cm) high to support and contain it.

Habitat and growth pattern

As it matures, the colorful untidy head develops tiny parachutelike seeds instead of each slim yellow petal. These can be easily blown away by the lightest puff of wind.

A cut portion of the deep tap root can regenerate into a completely new plant, showing its immense vitality underground as well as overground. Dandelion multiplies abundantly, and "untidies" the best-kept immaculate lawns. It is an enemy to overformality.

Dandelion knows when to rest; when it is too hot it closes up its petals.

FOLKLORE AND USAGE

❁ Dandelion frees the bladder, releases toxins from the blood, and helps to disperse premenstrual tension. This edible medicine helps "the brain of the body," the liver, in its work, prevents the hardening of stones in the gall bladder, and dissolves warts. Dandelion tea can sometimes relieve stomach cramps. It is useful for releasing many kinds of congestion.

Key words

POSITIVE: *Freedom, effortless dynamic energy, body consciousness.*
NEGATIVE: *Perfectionism, physical tension, lack of awareness of body.*

Challenge

To become aware of how controlling attitudes and emotions cause hardening of the muscles and other body tissues.

AFFIRMATION
I am
freedom-loving.

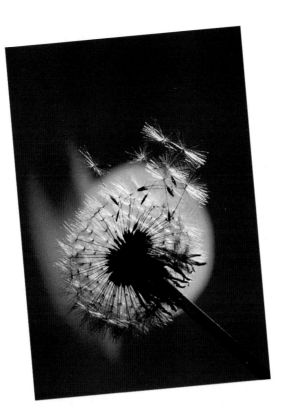

LEFT *The mature dandelion plant develops parachutelike seeds in place of its slender yellow petals.*

CASE STUDY

Justine, a very organized and busy working mother, age 40, took painkillers for her premenstrual pains so that she could continue being active. Rather than listen to her body's natural need to slow down for a while, she would rush around until she collapsed, sometimes with an incapacitating migraine. She began to take Dandelion essence and slowly came to understand how the painkillers might be contributing to her migraine. She became really enthused about free dancing. The more she danced, the more she was able to shake off her tension. Gradually she remembered in her childhood how her family believed the only legitimate reason for resting was illness. She began to see that there were times when she needed to slow down. After six months, she became free of premenstrual tension and migraines.

NOTES

Therapeutic actions
Helps the overactive person to relax; helps in understanding and expressing the causes of many otherwise mysterious aches and pains; supplemented by an oil or cream, it induces the body to relax and let go of muscle tension.

Method of making essence
Sun method; sun infusion of the flowers in oil.

Ways of using and use in combination
Massage oil; ointment; dosage bottle; bath.

Best supportive technique
Body awareness; massage; expressive dancing or any free movement; body psychotherapy; aromatherapy.

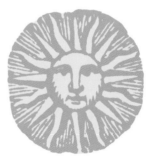

ABOVE *The dandelion is a flower of the sun and should be prepared by infusing the flowers in oil.*

LEFT *Dandelion essence may be added to massage oil to alleviate tension and aid relaxation.*

Thymus vulgaris

Thyme

THYME *is a fragrant aromatic herb of the mint family. This large group contains the most useful plants in nature's medicine chest. This family grows prolifically throughout the whole of Europe and Asia. Thyme particularly likes the hot sun of the Mediterranean where it is found on stony soils and dry grassland, scenting the air for miles around.*

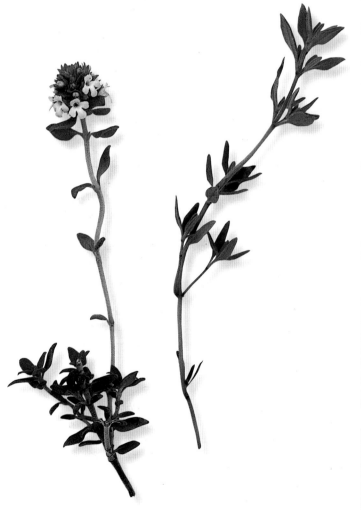

ABOVE *Common thyme has pale lilac flowers that appear in early midsummer.*

SIGNATURE

Fiery, grounded strength ensures health and achievement

Name
It is also called mother thyme, running thyme, and shepherd's thyme. Thyme is related to the Greek words *thuein*, to burn sacrifice, and *thymus*, meaning courage. *Thumos* also means "smell." Smell is connected strongly with animals marking out their territory to keep competitors at bay. *Vulgaris* means common. This, therefore, is a common thyme, an everyday way of keeping fear at bay.

Color/shape
The flowers are often reddish-purple and small but can come in many colors. The leaves are small with a spicy aroma. The flower is like an open mouth with fiercely protruding anthers, suggesting that it is warding off prey.

Habitat and growth pattern
Thyme is a bushy, cushionlike, spreading subshrub with hairy, aromatic gray-green leaves. The stems are highly branched and usually covered with small white hairs. In the wild it grows as an aromatic ground cover.

One of the main features of the mint family is its squarish stems. *Thymus vulgaris* has a square green-brown stem that becomes woody in the second year of growth. This gives it a greater earthiness than other varieties. Like other members of this family, thyme has four rows of leaves, and bears four seeds, representing solidity and protection.

It has smaller flowers than many other members of its family, which concentrates its energy into producing the antiseptic oil.

AFFIRMATION

I purify my motives that I may live without fear.

Key words
POSITIVE: *Protection, courage.*
NEGATIVE: *Viral infection, underachiever.*

Challenge
To become a warrior to find courage and the will to achieve goals.

FOLKLORE AND USAGE

❀ The Greeks spoke of smelling of thyme to imply that someone was brave, while Roman soldiers bathed in thyme water to give themselves vigor. In the Middle Ages, European ladies would embroider a handkerchief with sprig of thyme and a bee as inspiration for their knights.

❀ Wild thyme tea gave courage to the battling Highlanders of Scotland. Thyme's antiseptic and preservative powers mean that it has been useful to embalmers from Egyptian times until the present day. Its ability to kill microorganisms keep herbarium and anatomical specimens safe today from decay.

❀ According to folk magic, girls should wear a sprig of thyme, lavender, and mint to attract a sweetheart and

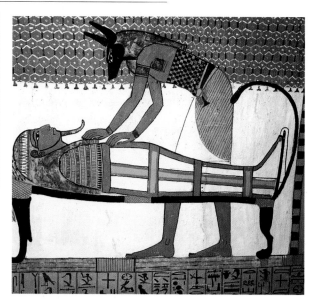

thyme on its own to attract the fairies.

❀ Thyme is used as a general tonic and to cure hangovers and nausea, among many others things. It produces an aromatic essential oil that is antiseptic, antiviral, and an immune stimulant.

ABOVE *Anubis, the god of embalmers, used medicinal herbs such as thyme as he prepared the dead for their journey to the underworld.*

The essential oil thymol can kill over 1,200 toxins that affect the body.

CASE STUDY

Tom was thinking of becoming self-employed after having been with the same company for a long time.
However, he imagined all the difficulties he would face if he set up his own company. While worrying about this he became ill with the flu. He was given Thyme essence and began to realize that he'd made himself ill with worry and that he needed time to sort himself out. He could see his father's face

laughing at him if he failed, and twisted with envy if he succeeded with the business.
After two days, he began to make a list of everything that needed attention and careful planning. He saw that his fears connected with his father were what he had to grapple with in himself and used the image of the open-mouthed thyme flower warriors scaring away his frightened boyhood memories of being mocked for the slightest failure. He realized that he wanted to

make his father jealous of him and that he had become so entangled in these thoughts that he had not been able to see the right way ahead.
Tom decided that all he really wanted was to earn a reasonable living and that it was worth going ahead with his plans. He felt that the Thyme essence had strengthened him by making him look at his motives honestly. He was then strong enough to make the break.

Valeriana officinalis

Valerian

VALERIAN *is a hardy, herbaceous perennial herb found throughout the world, except in Australasia. The valerian or* Valerianacea *family has 200 species that are native to Europe and northern Asia, and now naturalized to North America. They are extremely adaptable plants, growing in moist woodland, meadows, beside streams, or in rough, grassy, and bushy places. They also like mountainous regions, and the alpine species grow in scree or rock crevices. The dried root of the plant has a very distinctive smell and has been known to drive cats into a frenzy.*

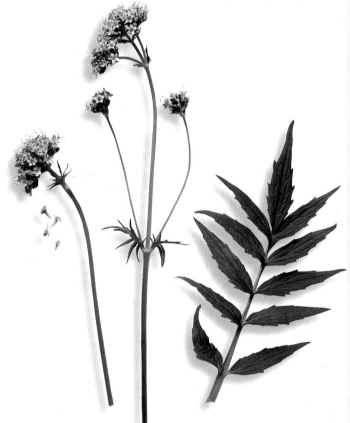

ABOVE *Small pinkish-white flowers appear on tall stems in midsummer.*

SIGNATURE

& *Provides deep nourishment to relax and calm us* &

Name
This plant is commonly called all heal or common valerian. Valerian is from the Latin verb *valere*, meaning to be healthy.

Color/shape
The flowers are very tiny, pale creamy to lavender pink, and grow in small clusters. Their smell is very peculiar, a bit like vanilla, and can be quite overwhelming. The narrow-toothed dark green leaflets also have a slightly unpleasant, sharp horseradish smell. Valerian can grow to 6ft. (2m) in height and 16–32in. (40–80cm) wide.

The flowers alone give very little evidence of their value. At first, they give the unattractive impression of people who don't feed themselves very well or take care of their personal hygiene. This impression is reinforced when we see that the stem too is skinny and anemic looking and is easily broken when young. The seeds are also light brown, flat, and poignantly tear-shaped.

Habitat and growth pattern
The dried root of valerian smells rancid, like stale perspiration. In fact, valeric acid is contained in human perspiration. The implication here is that too much hard work and not enough attention to emotional hygiene cripples the spirit.

There are sedative and rejuvenative properties to valerian's chemistry to counteract this sorry situation. The root is a short rhizome with pale fibrous offshoots. It has a strong effect on the earth surrounding it, stirring up phosphorus and creating rich compost.

Phosphorous glows in the dark and draws earthworms to it. So valerian root is as strong and lively as the valerian flower appears weak.

Valerian always remains free from pests and diseases in the garden, no doubt due to its unattractive smell, so it is able to keep harm away. It has the ability to generate numerous microspecies, and may be seen as encouraging us to find our own expression.

NOTES

Therapeutic actions
Alleviates stress, exhaustion, disturbed sleep and tension related to overwork; brings harmony in relationships through creating a greater sense of nourishment and support from within; opens up the joy and humor of the present moment; helps us reclaim our childhood right to just be and have fun, making us better companions to those we love.

Method of making essence
Sun method.

Ways of using and use in combination
Use with another essence that relaxes, such as Chamomile, and with Bush Gardenia to heal relationships.

Best supportive technique
Take time off work and give yourself a treat – go to a movie or take a refreshing walk.

Key words
POSITIVE: *Freedom, humor, spontaneity, warmth.*
NEGATIVE: *Weighed down by overwork, overadapted, relationship conflict.*

Challenge
To clear childhood trauma and to reclaim your right to enjoy life, and so find harmony in all your relationships.

FOLKLORE AND USAGE

❋ Nordic, Persian, and Chinese herbalists used valerian root medicinally. In Europe it has been used for hundreds of years as a remedy for nervous disorders, hysterical afflictions, and for epileptic attacks induced by strong emotions, such as anger and fear. In Britain, valerian was used during World Wars I and II to treat shell shock and to calm people after air raids.

❋ In herbalism today it is frequently used where there is pain connected with tension, such as migraine, and in orthodox medicine as a sedative. It is used in Germany today as a nerve tonic tea.

❋ Cats are attracted to the smell of valerian, reacting with intoxication. It could also have been what induced the rats of Hamelin to follow the Pied Piper.

❋ It is used to give a background to lighter, pleasanter smells to make a seductive perfume. Valerian was given to fighting couples to stop them from arguing. All this suggests the ability of valerian to bring relaxation and pleasure.

ABOVE *Cats are attracted to the musky smell of valerian root.*

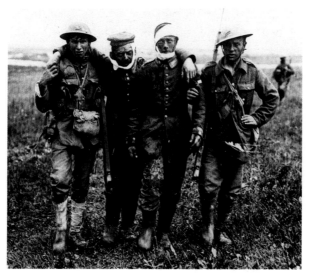

RIGHT *Valerian was used as a remedy for shell shock during World Wars I and II.*

CASE STUDY

Jennifer, a 35-year-old found herself unable to sleep. She was getting so impatient with her children that they were misbehaving in school. Her friends also complained that they never saw her. When she was given Valerian essence, Jennifer saw that she always caught up in her work as a hotelier. Although she still took care of her children physically, she realized that she had stopped enjoying them.

Jennifer remembered just how unplayful her own childhood had been. She was the oldest of five and always took care of her younger siblings while her parents were at work. She rarely played with children of her own age. Jennifer realized that she worked too hard because she didn't know how to play. With help from her friends, Jennifer began to join in walks and parties. She also started to enjoy her her children.

Verbascum thapsus

Mullein

MULLEIN *is a member of the foxglove* (Scrophulariaceae) *family, which includes* mimulus *and* calceolaria. *There are about 360 species of the* Verbascum, *which are cultivated because of their beautiful stateliness. In the wild they are found mainly on dry, stony hillsides, on wasteland, and in open woodland in places as far apart as Europe, North Africa, and west and central Asia. It is an abundant naturalized weed in eastern North America.*

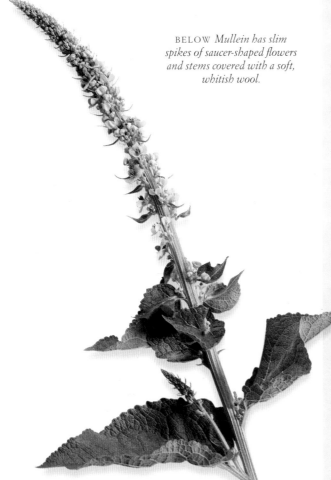

BELOW *Mullein has slim spikes of saucer-shaped flowers and stems covered with a soft, whitish wool.*

SIGNATURE

Be upright and softly cling to the truth so that your integrity shines

Name
Mullein is also known as king's truth, great mullein, poor man's flannel, hag's taper, hare's beard, Aaron's rod, and fairy's wand. Mullein derives from *mollis* **meaning soft.** *Verbascum* **is probably from** *barbascum*, **meaning a bearded plant.**

There are many folk names for mullein that go back to magical, mythical, and Christian history. It was named Aaron's rod after the Old Testament story concerning the rod of Levi on which Aaron's name was inscribed. This produced buds and blossoms when it was placed in the Tabernacle.

Color/shape
Mullein is a spectacular plant, upright and imposing, growing up to 6ft. (2m) in height.

The flowers are a warm yellow, which in heraldry signifies faith and constancy. As is often the case, a color can indicate the polarities of a quality, depending on circumstances and the exact shade and hue. Yellow can be used to mean treachery or cowardliness (as in "yellow-bellied") and Judas Iscariot is often portrayed in yellow garments in Christian art. However, at the same time St. Peter, for instance, who "holds the keys to heaven," is often shown wearing golden yellow garments.

Habitat and growth pattern
Mullein often grows on waste ground, where it will bloom over a long period of time. An angelic quality is evoked by the winglike upper leaves. In the same way, given time and support for the reclamation of the self, we can rise from dereliction to self-pride.

Mullein is very skillful in its use of moisture. Because of its tall spike, it is able to drop rain from its small leaves onto its larger leaves and down to the roots. The soft woolliness of the leaves cuts down water loss too. As well as using water efficiently, mullein's soft down keeps insects and grazing animals at bay because it irritates their mucous membranes.

FOLKLORE AND USAGE

AFFIRMATION

I am true to
my best self.

Key words

POSITIVE: *Truthfulness,
uprightness, conscience.*
NEGATIVE: *Self-deception,
tendency to lie, confusion.*

Challenge

*To tune into inner guidance
to live an upright life.*

NOTES

Therapeutic actions
*Helps us to listen
inwardly to ourselves;
helps develops
conscience and inner
morality; helps us to
develop an appropriate
awareness of where we
have gone wrong.*

**Method of
making essence**
*Sun method. Pick the
flowers only where there
is a good strong group of
mature, well-established
plants that can spare a
few blooms.*

**Ways of using and
use in combination**
*Good with Self-heal,
Amazon Waterlily, and
Sunflower.*

**Best supportive
technique**
*Confide truthfully in
someone you trust;
write a journal.*

❇ The leaves of mullein were traditionally used to line shoes to keep feet warm in the winter, and its soft fine hairs were used for tinder for making fires.

❇ In the epic story of Ulysses, Circe, a sorceress, turned Ulysses' companions into swine, but he was able to resist the spell because he was protected by mullein that had been given to him by the god Mercury. The power of mullein gave Ulysses integrity, helping him to resist being reduced to his "animal" nature.

❇ Mullein has long been used, literally, to light the way. The folk names "candlewick plant" and "high taper" refer to the fact that the "wool" was used for lamp wicks. The whole stem was dipped into fat or pitch and set alight to become a torch, taper, funeral candle, or a flare to shine from afar.

❇ In Ireland, mullein is considered as a specific for

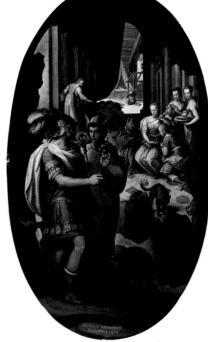

every kind of lung problem. It was even added to tobacco. As the tobacco damaged the lungs, so mullein helped them recover. It is still used today for poultices.

ABOVE *Mullein gave Ulysses
protection against the evil
powers of the sorceress Circe.*

❇ Mullein's dried flowers can be used to treat bronchitis, colds, coughs, and hayfever. The flowers used to be steeped in hot water and drunk to relieve coughs, respiratory mucous, and hoarseness. Mullein flowers steeped in olive oil are excellent for easing ear problems. Thus mullein breaks down barriers to breathing freely and softens that which stops us from listening to ourselves.

CASE STUDY

William, in his 30s, was a divorcee who shared custody of his two young sons with his wife. William found that taking care of the boys was more difficult than he had expected. He asked his girlfriend to help, although he still had hopes of a reconciliation with his ex-wife. William started taking Mullein. His conscience began to trouble him and he started to be more truthful with the women in his life. A new honest relationship was established with both his wife and girlfriend.

Victoria amazonica or regia

Amazon Waterlily

T HE NYMPHAEACEAE *is the family of water plants to which the Amazon waterlily belongs. The family also includes other waterlilies and the sacred lotus. The family is found throughout the world in ponds, streams, and lakes.* Victoria Amazonica *is one of two species of deep-water plants occurring in tropical South America in the slow-moving backwaters of the Amazon.*

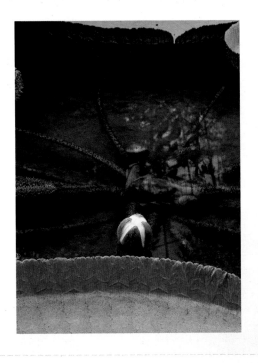

ABOVE *The Amazon waterlily is the largest of the waterlilies, growing up to 1ft. (30cm) across.*

SIGNATURE

❦ *Wisdom ripens through proper spiritual discipline* ❧

Name

This plant is also known as the giant waterlily, royal waterlily, or Queen Victoria waterlily. The family of waterlilies, the *Nymphea*, take their name from the Greek water deity, *Nymphe*, the goddess of springs and a guardian of nature. This one is not only a goddess but also a queen.

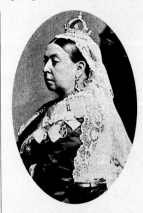

ABOVE *The Amazon waterlily is also known as the Queen Victoria waterlily.*

Color/shape

Amazon lilies are spectacular to behold. They grow from stout rhizomes buried deep in the bed of the river or pool. In the summer, they bear many-petaled, night-blooming white flowers. The sepals of the flower are prickly. The flowers change rapidly from white to purplish-red on the day on which they come to maturation. White is the color of transcendence, the capacity to go beyond the physical world, and the purplish-red is at the opposite end of the spectrum, helping us to live life actively with all our senses.

Habitat and growth pattern

The single leaf grows to 6ft. (2m) in diameter with a vertical rim all around the edge between 4in. (10cm) or, occasionally, 6in. (15cm) high.

The leaf looks like an enormous round tray sitting on top of the water. It is midgreen with prickles all over and reddish-purple underneath. Both the flower and the leaves rest gracefully on top of the water. The waterlily's stalk has to be very strong to support the weight of both flower and leaf.

The circle has always represented perfection, and in nature the role of the leaf is to keep the balance between the intake and elimination of gases. The rim of the waterlily leaf suggests protection, and the prickles of the sepals and the leaf help keep intruders at bay.

Even in cultivation, this plant remains pest-free, which reinforces its association with strength and purity.

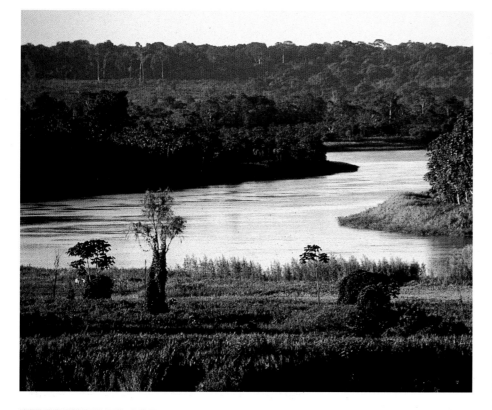

AFFIRMATION
I am attaining superb physical emotional and spiritual well-being.

Key words

POSITIVE: *Balance and grace, eternal youth.*
NEGATIVE: *Physical neglect, aging, death.*

Challenge

To cherish your body as a sacred vehicle for your mind and soul.

CASE STUDY

Ann, in her late 50s, was extremely exhausted and felt depressed and extremely apathetic. After taking Amazon Waterlily, Ann began to feel more energetic. A week later, she decided to join a yoga class, and also began to follow a macrobiotic diet. A month later, Ann was feeling very good about her body and found herself wanting to have private times for contemplation. She felt she had regained her dignity as a human being. A month later, she joined a meditation class. She had not only regained her balance and energy, she was beginning to experience states of bliss.

NOTES

Therapeutic actions

Acts as a real tonic to the subtle energy systems of the body; it uplifts the emotions and heightens awareness by increasing energy through the outer membrane of the spine and the flow of nerve fluid (this brings an added vitality that strengthens the ability to take a long view and release oneself from negative emotions); brings a powerful release of natural energy into the body that can support the transformational process of dying and physiological death.

Method of making essence.

Crystal method. Refer to Andreas Korte's book (see Bibliography pp. 140-141).

Ways of using and use in combination

Use after solving or coming to terms with emotional issues; best taken alone for a time in a dosage bottle or with Ruby gem elixir.

Best supportive technique

Patchouli oil to clarify problems and as a tonic; hatha yoga; vegetarian diet; read the teachings of sages, such as "The Tibetan Book of Living and Dying."

ABOVE *The Amazon waterlily can be found growing in the tributaries of the great Amazon River that runs through tropical South America.*

FOLKLORE AND USAGE

❀ Like the lotus flower, the waterlily is traditional associated with the working of spirit on matter. Growing rooted deep in the mud, rising up through the water, and floating above it, breathing in the fresh air and sunlight, it represents the human body as a vehicle that can transmute matter into pure spirit.

Zinnia elegans
Zinnia

ZINNIA *is a member of the largest family of all plants – the sunflower family. There are around 20 species that all enjoy the dry, hot summers of Mexico. They also grow well in the southwestern states of the United States, South and Central America. It likes these sunny locations, but also needs rich, fertile soil. It blooms happily from summer through to winter. There is a larger version of Zinnia elegans, Zinnia grandiflora or Prairie Zinnia, which was used by the Zuni Indians of South America to cure fever. The whole plant was powdered and sprinkled over hot stones and the fumes were then inhaled by the patient.*

BELOW *The central disk and radiating petals look like a wide open-eye with lashes.*

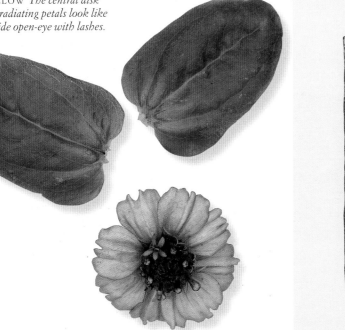

SIGNATURE

❧ *Playfulness relieves overseriousness* ❧

Name
Zinnia is like the word zany. *Elegans* means elegant, so it could be taken to mean beautifully humorous!

Color/shape
The daisylike flowers come in a huge variety of colors, but are mainly white, yellow, orange, crimson, red, purple, or lilac, some with white eyes. The most potent flower for an essence is probably the bright red variety, the color that children are most often drawn to. This plant comes from Mexico, which is famous for the richness of color of its carnivals and its joyous fiestas. Zinnia helps us to come into contact with the simplicity of our child nature.

Habitat and growth pattern
Zinnia is an ornamental plant with many brightly colorful hybrids. They come in a variety of forms too – as erect annuals, perennials, and small shrubs – and are very resistant to pests and diseases. So they give themselves plenty of creative freedom and stay strong in the process.

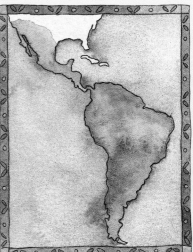

ABOVE *The zinnia species flourishes in the climates of the southern United States, Central and South America.*

Key words

POSITIVE: *Good humor,
playfulness, generosity,
light-heartedness.*
NEGATIVE: *Overserious,
devitalized, deprived
inner child.*

Challenge

*To release emotional and
mental toxicity through
playfulness so that you can
freely give and receive love.*

NOTES

Therapeutic actions
*Zinnia works on the part of
the brain that deals with
unlearned, pre-programed
behavior. When this part of
the brain is dominant we
can become overaggressive
or submissive. Our fears,
anxieties, insecurities, and
exhaustion rule us and we
become critical and dull.
Zinnia sensitizes us to
recognizing the nurturing
that already exists for us in
our environment. This
helps us to release feelings
of bitterness and returns us
to good humor.*

**Method of
making essence**
Sun method.

**Ways of using and
use in combination**
*Use in a dosage bottle;
place two drops directly
onto unbroken skin and
rub in; use with Chamomile
and/or Valerian.*

Best supportive technique
*Tissue salts of Nat. phos.,
Ferr. phos., and Nat. mur.
are very useful; enjoying
comedy of any sort; playing
with children.*

CASE STUDY

**Sarah, a 40-year-old
mature student, had
been having counseling
to deal with the abuse
that she had suffered
during her childhood.**
She had learned to be
angry with, rather than
feel victimized by, her
attackers, and her
therapy appeared to be
going well. However,
she had become angry
and suspicious of the
people around her, and
oversensitive to the
slightest hint of being
"put down." After
taking Zinnia for one
week, she felt a lot more
relaxed with everyone
around her and was
even told that her
humor had lightened an
overserious class.

Another example of
the effects of Zinnia
concerns 70-year-old
Joyce who was suffering
from a neurological
disease. Her illness
affected her brain in
such a way that she was
always irritable.
However, taking Zinnia
for a couple of months
brought out a very
pleasant personality.
Eventually she no
longer needed to take
Zinnia to help her be
positive and cheerful.

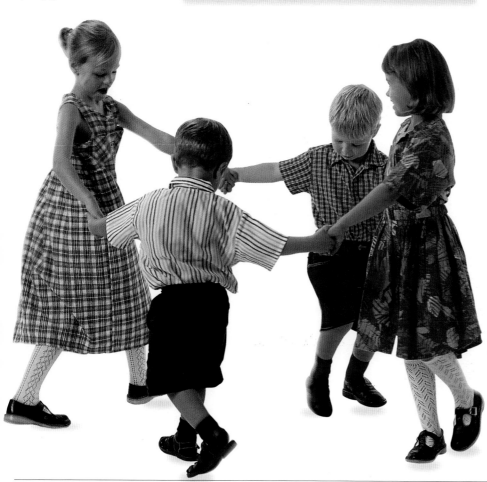

LEFT *The center of the
zinnia plant contains an
irregular crown of starlike
yellow anthers, like children
dancing in a circle.*

Supportive Techniques

IN WORKING WITH *ourselves or our clients it is important to be to able understand ways of following through the healing impulses generated by flower essences. They can't do everything. This section includes only a few of the possible ways in which we may consolidate the gains we have made in taking essences so that they may become permanent. If you are a flower essence practitioner or counselor it is very important to be able to recognize your limitations and refer on.*

Acupressure and Shiatsu

Acupressure is a development from acupuncture using the fingers rather than needles, to stimulate or tone the flow of energy through the meridians or energy (*chi*) channels in the body. Shiatsu, which is Japanese for "finger pressure," is the Japanese development of this technique. It uses the same meridians and pressure points but has different techniques to stimulate them. It is both a treatment and a system of self-help.

Affirmations

Affirmations work to support the cognitive level of change. Words are articulated in a way that actively help to reframe, with positive intent, negative beliefs about ourselves or others. Experimenting with affirmations usually brings subconscious beliefs to the surface enabling us to shed their undermining influences. It is important to find supportive ways to release the suppressed feelings, held tensions, and blockages in the body that hold these negative beliefs in place.

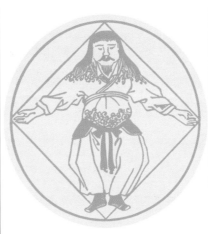

ABOVE *Many of the supportive techniques originate in other cultures, or countries such as Japan.*

Aromatherapy

The healing properties of aromatic oils extracted from plants such as rose or lavender have been utilized for at least the last 5,000 years. Beautiful fragrances have a powerful ability to influence our mood. Each essential oil has different properties; some are stimulating while others are relaxing. In aromatherapy massage, these oils are used in a "carrier" oil such as avocado or almond, and their various healing properties are assimilated directly into the bloodstream.

Awareness techniques

In order to develop awareness we have to practice bringing our attention to our own unique ongoing experiences of being "within" a body and in the world. This form of therapy involves staying in the present by noticing what we are sensing, feeling, touching, hearing, visualizing, thinking, or seeing and enables us to literally "come to our senses." Awareness techniques can focus on inner or outer experiences.

Biodynamic therapy

This form of therapy seeks to enhance the free flow of energy in the body. It is based on the awareness that disruptions to the flow of our biological energy occur when, instead of finding ways to express our feelings, we repress important emotions. This repression causes tension and disease. The biodynamic therapist uses massage and body movement, together with counseling, to help clients to come to terms with their emotions and recognize what they are feeling, then find the appropriate means of expression to address this.

Body awareness
or sensory awareness

 This was developed by Charlotte Selver out of work by Elsa Ginder. Ginder suffered from tuberculosis but, by becoming so sensitive to the workings of her body and nervous system, she was able to allow the diseased lung to rest and so cure herself of the disease. Frits Parls, the Berlin psychoanalyst and founder of Gestalt therapy, was highly influenced by her work.

Counseling

A trained counselor will support his or her clients in adjusting to the various life problems that may be causing them great distress. He or she will teach their clients a way of learning to cope with such problems. The counselor helps clients to make changes in attitude that will lead them to take action to relieve or reduce their discomfort so that they may enjoy health and happiness. Many different techniques are used including Rogerian therapy, neurolinguistic programing, and Gestalt therapy.

Craniosacral therapy

A craniosacral practitioner will tune into the subtle movements of the bones and membranes of the skull and the sacrum with his or her hands. Freeing blockages in the cranial movement increases the health of the central nervous system itself, thus increasing the body's ability to find balance and respond more healthily to disease.

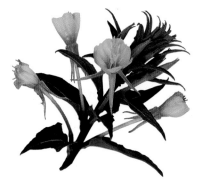

ABOVE *The oil of the Evening Primrose makes an excellent carrier oil for use in aromatherapy.*

Creative visualization

This uses the power of the imagination to release dormant imagery within the psyche for healing and extending consciousness. Imagination has a powerful influence on our body and mind. Guided visualization can support the imagination to amplify different layers of consciousness. Active imagination can be used to extend our access to the unconscious and help us to bring dream material to successful completion.

Crystal therapy

 Crystals, semiprecious stones, and gems – these are mineral blossoms of the earth. They have been used and revered since the dawning of civilization as sources of earthly light. The clear quartzes, which include amethyst and citrine, are commonly called crystals. Semiprecious stones and gems include emerald, ruby, sapphire, and turquoise. They are often used with flower essences to ground and amplify them. See books by Alaskan Flower Essence Project and Andreas Korte (*see Bibliography pp. 140–141*).

Dowsing

 Dowsing is used by many flower essence practitioners and makers to find the appropriate flower essences for a client. For this you need a pendulum and your essences handy. You can make a pendulum yourself by attaching a suitable object to a piece of string, so that it swings freely.

Find out which way the pendulum swings when you say "no" to it, and which way it goes when you say "yes". A rapid circling motion often means yes, and a side-to-side movement no. Establish your own code to find out which essences are appropriate to your needs.

It is generally easier to dowse for another person, especially if he or she is not known to you. There are many ways in which the pendulum's movement can be influenced, so bear in mind that your answers may not always be as reliable as you would wish. You can use the "answer" as a stimulus to thinking. You can always find ways of checking your results through other techniques, including listening to feedback from the person for whom you are dowsing.

Five rhythms dancing

Discovered by Gabriel Roth, these rhythms are five natural rhythms in the body that roughly correlate to the five elements. You are free to explore any movement that feels good to you in response to the music based on these beats. It is very powerful in releasing stagnant energy in the body and enlivening your energy in a balanced and enjoyable way.

Focusing

 Eugene Gendlin, a professor of psychology, conducted an investigation to determine what the most proficient psychotherapists did with their clients. He discovered it was the therapists' support of a natural process, which he called focusing, that enabled clients to connect their awareness to body experiences. He made it into a teachable technique called focusing.

Gestalt therapy

 This therapy takes its name from a psychological theory of perception that says we are continually seeking to make wholes or "gestalts" at all levels of our experience. Gestalt therapists therefore guide their clients, using various techniques, which bring them into the fullest awareness in the present. This enables them to experience how they construct their lives instead of focusing on the why.

Hatha yoga

Ha means sun and *tha* means moon. Hatha yoga can be understood as the integration of opposite aspects of the person, including right and left sides of the body and mind. It is the most commonly known aspect of the yoga system and includes *pranayama* – breathing techniques and *asanas* – stretching postures; these include the cobra, the plow, and the tree.

RIGHT *Crystal therapy can be used in conjunction with flower essence therapy to enhance its healing power.*

Homeopathy

 Homeopathy comes from *homios* meaning "same" and *patos,* which means "suffering." A homeopathic remedy produces the same symptoms in a healthy person as those exhibited by the sick person, that is "like cures like." This is contrasted with allopathic medicine where disease is generally treated by attacking or counteracting the disease.

Muscle testing

Muscle testing is sometimes called applied kinesiology. This can be used very simply or in an extremely sophisticated way in relation to the meridian system. Machaelle Small Wright of Perelandra Essences has a wonderful way of using muscle testing for assessing which remedies to use (*see Bibliography pp. 140–1*).

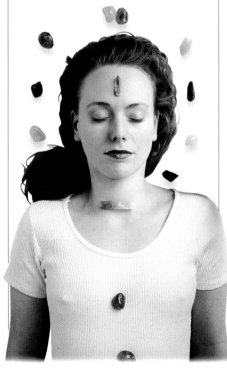

New floral remedies

There are some exciting developments within flower essence therapy, utilizing knowledge of their energy flows.

• Based upon traditional acupuncture points, Drs. Vasudeva and Kadambii Barnao have developed floral acu maps, which indicate where to use their special creams and remedies. Refer to these in their "Walkabout Healing Handbook" (*see Bibliography pp. 140–141.*)

• A very potent way of using the Bach Flower Remedies is given in "New Bach Flower Body Maps, Treatment by Topical Application." Sore body parts are also used as a means of diagnosing which particular Bach Flower Remedy is appropriate.

• The Flower Essence Society of California has developed some wonderful combined flower essences and aromatherapy oils. These are very powerful because they utilize the physical properties of oils as they permeate the body via the skin, the aromas, influence on the brain via the olfactory glands, together with the subtle properties of the flower essence taken up by the vibrational bodies.

NLP or neurolinguistic programing

This is a body of theory derived from systematically analyzing exceptional people and experiences to enable others to benefit. A major aspect of neurolinguistic programing therapy is to help clients to reprogram or reframe experiences in a way that optimizes their chances for happiness and success.

Osteopathy

Once regarded as an alternative therapy, osteopathy has become part of orthodox medical treatment in many countries, including the United States. Osteopathy comes from the Greek *osteos* "bone" and *pathos* "disease." Osteopaths manipulate the body's structure in an effort to restore general health. It is based on the theory that disease is due chiefly to mechanical derangement of the tissues, with special emphasis on restoring the structural integrity of the spine through manipulation.

Polarity therapy

This is a holistic healing system. It aims to balance the energy circuits of the body through diet, touch, exercise, and attitude. From an integrated theoretical and practical base the therapist uses knowledge and techniques of touch that are known as the separate techniques of craniosacral therapy, acupressure, osteopathy, and reflexology.

Psychotherapy

Psychotherapy can, in practice, overlap with counseling, but its emphasis is on the exploration over time of the process that causes distress. Problems are explored in depth, in terms of their meaning and significance in the overall life pattern of the client. The aim of neurolinguistic therapy is self-renewal from actively understanding and making the most of psychological resources.

Radionics

Invented in the 1920s by an American, Albert Abrams, this technique involves healing at a distance with the aid of a special radionic instrument, a "mysterious black box." Before commencing treatment with the box, the practitioner will ask the client for a "witness," such as a lock of hair or a drop of blood, which is then used for diagnostic purposes. The radionics practitioner may also recommend that his or her client uses flower essences or homeopathic medicines.

Reiki

This system of healing evolved from the experience and dedication of a Japanese minister, Dr. Mikao Usui, in the late 19th century. "Reiki" means "universal life energy" in the Japanese language. Reiki practitioners are attuned to energy that enables them to treat themselves and other people through a series of hand positions. This usually produces a profound state of relaxation that revitalizes and balances the body, supporting the patients' natural ability to heal themselves.

Rogerian therapy

Rogerian therapy is the most common basic training for counselors worldwide. Therapists are trained to develop attitudes of completely respecting, empathically understanding, and being real with their clients. This melts any defenses created by harsh parenting, and empowers the client to apply these attitudes to themselves.

Tissue salts

Dr. Schussler (1821–98) believed that all diseases result from a imbalance of one or more of the 12 basic tissue salts. One salt is Nat. phos. or Naturum phosphoricum, which is commonly called phosphate of soda, and regulates the acid level in the cells. These salts could be used for indigestion, nausea, or heartburn, and can be found in most health food stores.

Vibrational

Medical practitioners often use a vega machine. This is based on the principle of electrical resistance matching the energy from an essence to the energy from a person. Most often acupuncture points are tested. When there is a match to the right essence, the machine makes a noise. Arthur Bailey has written a very thorough book on these and many other aspects of dowsing (*see Bibliography pp. 140–1*).

Yoga

The word yoga means "to yoke" or "to join." The ultimate yogic aim is to enable the practitioner to attain enlightenment, to rejoin the soul with the Supreme Being. To achieve this, yogis use the eight limbs of this system of self-transformation. They are *yama* – abstinence; *niyama* – cultivation of purity; *asana* – physical posture; *pranayama* – breath control; *pratyahara* – nondistraction; *dharana* – concentration; *dhyana* – contemplation or meditation; *samadhi* – bliss of union.

Combining and Combinations

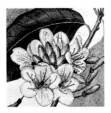

ABOVE *One of the ingredients of Bach's Rescue Remedy is Rock Rose.*

MANY MODERN *flower essence-makers combine different essences to make a synergistic formula, one in which the whole is greater than the sum of the parts. Some combination essences have a single essence combined with plant essential oils or tinctures synergistically. Read up about aromatherapy essential oils and their properties and try making your own formulas. By obtaining the maker's literature you will find out the full range of formulas available to you.*

The following list includes all the composite formulas mentioned in this book. However, not all the flowers in each combination are covered in this book. If you want to make them up for yourself, look in Useful Addresses (*see p. 139*) for the essence maker or distributor. They will generally supply the individual flower essences singly, for you to combine yourself.

Rescue Remedy
• *Bach Flower Remedies.*
Bach discovered a combination he called Rescue Remedy. Called the 39th remedy, it is made with five flowers and has been used all over the world for many years to help in all kinds of emergencies. Every temperament will find in this remedy a flower that suits their major response to shock.

Dandelion Oil
• *The Flower Essence Society of California,* (F.E.S.).
This is a great massage oil, and is especially useful for unknotting tight muscles and easing painful menstrual cramps. It is wonderful for use in the bath too. It is made from a base of olive oil, rosemary oil, castor oil, Dandelion essence, and herb tincture.

THE FIVE FLOWERS OF DR. BACH'S RESCUE REMEDY

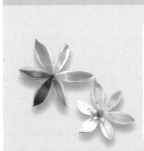 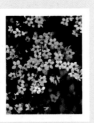 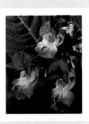 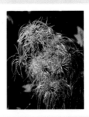 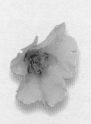

Star of Bethlehem
for consolation after shock.

Cherry Plum
for fear of losing control.

Impatiens
for mental agitation.

Clematis
for dreaminess, since many people respond to an emergency by cutting out.

Rock Rose
for courage to face an emergency.

Dynamis Essence

• *Bush Essences.*

This helps recover our drive and enthusiasm and harmonizes our vital forces when we have been ill. It consists of Old Man Banksia, *Macrocarpa*, Crowea, Wild Potato Bush, and *Banskia Robur.*

Immune Formula

• *Desert Alchemy.*

This works to strengthen our protective systems through becoming aware of our own boundaries and individuality. It contains Bougainvillea, Fire Prickly Pear Cactus, Foothills Paloverde, Klein's Pencil Cholla Cactus, and Smartweed.

Meditation Essence

• *Bush Essences.*

This awakens spirituality. It is made from Fringed Violet, Bush Fuchsia, Bush Iris, Angelsword, and Red Lily.

Pain Cream and Arthritis Cream

• *Living Essences.*

These are made for the painful and stiff joints caused by rheumatism and arthritis, and for pain relief, including bruises, cramp, menstrual discomfort, and sinus pain. They are made from a selection of native Australian essences that have been researched over 12 years.

Relationship Essence

• *Bush Essences.*

This essence will clear away early negative conditioning patterns that interfere with harmony in intimate relationships. It consists of Bluebell, Bush Gardenia, Dagger Hakea, Mint Bush, Red Suva Frangipani, Boab, and Flannel Flower.

MAKING YOUR OWN COMBINATIONS

An infinite variety of situations can be faced with the 49 essences we feature here. While the essences are very effective used singly, combinations have the added advantage of taking care of many aspects of a problem at one time. The most effective combinations work to cover different responses to the same problem. To determine the right combination for your needs, use the following procedure.

Decide what issue is most important for you, then use the indexes (*see pp.127–135*) to help you find the appropriate essence for the issue, then read the pages devoted to that particular flower.

Refocus and ask yourself what else you need to cover. Repeat the procedure until you feel satisfied with the combination – this in itself is part of the healing process. If you have chosen the right flowers, you will begin to feel it even before you take the essence because you will have been impacted by the positive thoughts connected to those plants. However, it is important to note that the flowers, although harmless, have active properties that will start to awaken your mind, so don't stimulate too many themes at once. You can use up to five flowers at one time without getting too complex, but the simpler the better.

Self-heal Cream

• *The Flower Essence Society of California, (F.E.S.).*

This is a very effective natural skincare balm and first aid support. It is made from Self-heal, fresh plant tincture and essence, comfrey extract, and avocado oil.

St. John's Wort Oil

• *The Flower Essence Society of California, (F.E.S.).*

This is an excellent sunscreen and an effective remedy for wounds. It helps those people who do not feel that they are quite in their bodies to become grounded. Use this oil in the bath or apply it directly. It may be diluted further with other oils. The St. John's Wort flowers are sun-infused in olive oil, to which is added St. John's Wort flower essence together with angelica essential oil.

Single Mothers' Formula

• *Desert Alchemy.*

Made from Fairy Duster and Wild Sunflower, it deals with feeling physically and emotionally overwhelmed.

Travel Essence

• *Bush Essences.*

This helps travelers to arrive at their destination refreshed. It contains *Banksia Robur*, Bush Iris, Bottlebrush, Bush Fuchsia, Crowea, Fringed Violet, *Macrocarpa*, *Mulla Mulla*, Paw Paw, She Oak, and Sundew.

Yarrow Special Formula

• *The Flower Essence Society of California, (F.E.S.).*

A good tonic to combat the harsh technological and environmental challenges of the modern world. It consists of Yarrow, Echinacea, and Arnica in a sea salt water base.

Essence-makers

MANY ESSENCE-MAKERS *use the same flowers in their repertories. However, the healing effect of the flower essence will be related to the qualities of the environment and the mental attitude of the flower essence-maker. Flower essence-makers also use different techniques that bring out varying qualities of the plant. If you live in Britain you might buy Yarrow from Harebell in Scotland rather than from the Flower Essence Society of California, known as F.E.S., but of course the choice is yours.*

ABOVE *Borage essence can be bought from F.E.S.*

Amazon Waterlily, *Victoria amazonica*
Andreas Korte

Apple, *Malus sylvestris var. domestica*
Master's Flower Essences

Ash, *Fraxinus excelsior*
Green Man Tree Essences

Black Kangaroo Paw, *Macrophidia fuliginosa* Living Essences

Bleeding Heart, *Dicentra formsa*
Andreas Korte, Deva, F. E. S.

Borage, *Borago officinalis*
Andreas Korte, Deva, Dutch Flower Essences, F. E. S., Harebell Remedies

Bougainvillea, *Bougainvillea spectabilis*
Desert Alchemy, Hawaiian Tropical Flower Essences, Petite Fleur

Bush Gardenia, *Gardenia megasperma*
Bush Essences

Chamomile, *Anthemis nobilis*
F. E. S.

Cherry Plum, *Prunus cerasifera*
Bach Flower Remedies, Healing Herbs

Chicory, *Cicorium intybus*
Bach Flower Remedies, Healing Herbs

Clematis, *Clematis vitalba*
Bach Flower Remedies, Healing Herbs, Dutch Flower Remedies

Crab Apple, *Malus sylvestris*
Bach Flower Remedies, Healing Herbs

Crowea, *Crowea saligna*
Bush Essences

Dampiera, *Dampiera linearis*
Living Essences

Dandelion, *Taraxacum officinale*
Alaskan Flower Essence Project, Andreas Korte, Deva, F. E. S., Harebell Remedies, New Perception Flower Essences

Evening Primrose, *Oenothera hookeri*
Dutch Flower Essences, F. E. S., New Perception Flower Essences

Fairy Duster, *Calliandra eriophylla*
Desert Alchemy

Fireweed, *Epilobium angustifolium*
Alaskan Flower Essence Project, Deva, Pacific Essences

Garlic, *Allium sativum*
F. E. S.

Himalayan Slipper Orchid, *Paphiodilum insigne* Andreas Korte

Holly, *ilex aquifolium*
Bach Flower Remedies, Healing Herbs

Honesty, *Lunaria annua*
Dutch Flower Essences

Impatiens, *Impatiens glandulifera*
Bach Flower Remedies, Healing Herbs

Larch, *Larix decidua*
Bach Flower Remedies, Healing Herbs

Lilac, *Syringa vulgaris*
Alaskan Flower Essence Project, Bailey Essences, Deva, Green Man Tree Essences, Harebell Remedies, Petite Fleur

Macrozamia, *Macrozamia reidleii*
Living Essences

Madia, *Madia elegans*
F. E. S.

Menzies Banksia, *Banksia menziesii*
Living Essences

Mullein, *Verbascum thapsus*
Andreas Korte, Desert Alchemy, Deva, F. E. S.

Oak, *Quercus robur*
Bach Flower Remedies, Healing Herbs

Olive, *Olea europoea*
Bach Flower Remedies, Healing Herbs

Rock Rose, *Helianthemum nummularium*
Bach Flower Remedies, Healing Herbs

St. John's Wort, *Hypericum perforatum*
F. E. S.

Sea Anemone, *Anthopleura elegantissima*
Pacific Essences

Self-heal, *Prunella vulgaris*
Andreas Korte, Deva, F. E. S., Harebell Remedies

She Oak, *Casuarina glauca*
Bush Essences

Silver Princess, *Eucalyptus caesis*
Bush Essences, Living Essences

Star of Bethlehem, *Ornithogalum umbellatum* Bach Flower Remedies, Healing Herbs

Sticky Geranium, *Geranium erianthum*
Alaskan Flower Essence Project.

Sunflower, *Helianthus annuus*
Alaskan Flower Essence Project, Andreas Korte, Deva, F. E. S., Harebell Remedies, New Perception Essences, Petite Fleur

Thyme, *Thymus vulgaris*
Petite Fleur

Valerian, *Valeriana officinalis*
Andreas Korte, Bailey Essences, Desert Alchemy, Deva, Findhorn Essences, New Perception Essences

Walnut, *Juglans regia*
Bach Flower Remedies, Healing Herbs

Wild Oat, *Bromus ramosus*
Bach Flower Remedies, Healing Herbs

Wild Potato Bush, *Solanum quadriloculatum*
Bush Essences

Wild Rose, *Rosa canina*
Bach Flower Remedies, Healing Herbs

Yarrow, *Achillea millefolium*
Alaskan Flower Essence Project, F. E. S., Harebell Remedies

Zinnia, *Zinnia elegans*
Andreas Korte, Deva, F. E. S., Petite Fleur, Perelandra

Emergency Essences Index

DR. BACH'S *Rescue Remedy or Healing Herbs' Five Flower Formula are regarded as two of the best-known combinations for use in emergencies* (see p. 124). *The following list includes single essences and combinations from all over the world that can help to reduce stress in times of crisis. Where an essence made by a specific essence-maker is recommended, it is listed after each essence.*

Accidents and emergencies, of every kind:
Five Flower Formula [Healing Herbs], Rescue Remedy [Bach Flower Remedies]

Balance during shocks about health:
Crowea [Bush Essences], Self-heal [F.E.S.]

Conflict resolving:
Holly [Bach Flower Remedies]

Crisis and opportunity:
Desert Emergency Formula (Aloe Vera, Cliff Fendlerbush, Desert Holly, Klein's Pencil Cholla, and Purple Aster) [Desert Alchemy]

Earthquake:
Rescue Remedy [Bach Flower Remedies]

Emotional emergency, due to urgent need for change:
Fireweed Combo (Dwarf Fireweed, Fireweed, River Beauty, White Fireweed) [Alaskan Flower Essence Project]

First aid, an emergency combination that clears blockages and gives strength in difficult circumstances:
Terra (Angelica, Clematis, Mycena, Orchid, Yellow Star Tulip) [Dutch Flower Essences]

Grounding after shock:
Clematis [Bach Flower Remedies], Fireweed [Alaskan Flower Essence Project]

Headache:
Dampiera, Impatiens

Mental states needing release:
Dampiera

Nervous breakdown:
Dampiera [Living Essences], Rock Rose [Bach Flower Remedies], Fairy Duster [Desert Alchemy]

Old issues that prevent us from dealing with current crisis:
Trauma Remedy (Blackthorn, Celandine, Nettle, Butterbur, Daisy, and Primrose) [Unitive Flower and Life Essences]

Pain in shock:
Fireweed [The Alaskan Flower Project], and Sea Anemone [Pacific Essences]

Pain:
Menzies Banksia, Dampiera, Pain Cream [Living Essences], Sea Anemone [Pacific Essences]

Panic:
Emergency Essence (Fringed Violet, Gray Spider Flower, Sundew, Waratah, and Crowea) [Bush Essences], Rock Rose [Bach Flower Remedies]

Physical trauma:
Bluebell, Chamomile, Comfrey, and Red Clover essences [Harebell Remedies] (this is very good after injury or operation; works well with animals and children)

Post-trauma, for dealing with the after-effects:
a blend of Hibiscus, Impatiens, Noni, Dill, Potato, Four o'clock [Hawaiian Tropical Flower Essences]

Psychic protection:
Walnut [Bach Flower Remedies], Yarrow [F.E.S.]

Stress release:
Lavender, Red Clover, Sage, Self-heal, and Yarrow [Harebell Remedies] (this can be used to steady the nerves when feeling stressed or as a course of treatment for the nervous system)

Suicidal:
Cherry Plum [Bach Flower Remedies]

Surgery:
Rescue Remedy [Bach Flower Remedies]

Taking charge, during emergency:
Cherry Plum

Thought or fear of shock:
Star of Bethlehem, Impatiens [Bach Flower Remedies]

Unwinding after shock:
Star of Bethlehem, Impatiens [Bach Flower Remedies]

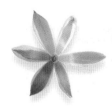

ABOVE *Star of Bethlehem is one of the best remedies to use for unwinding after a shock.*

Life Cycle Index

YOU CAN USE *flower essences to support you and your family throughout your life.*
The essences can enhance and enrich your natural cycles of experience and help you
through both the minor and major crises of life. Remember too that you may have
had challenging or damaging experiences at some point in your life that have remained
with you, unresolved and interfering with your ability to respond to the present.
If this is the case, you can use the life cycle index below to help you heal retrospectively.
If you feel you are particularly drawn to doing this, it is also advisable to
seek help from a competent counselor or therapist.

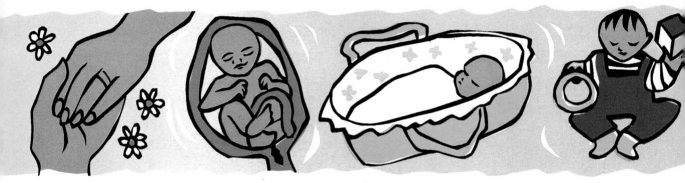

CONCEPTION
Problems with fertility:
She Oak

PREGNANCY
Absorption of toxic
emotions by child:
Evening Primrose
Cheerful anticipation:
Borage
Deciding whether to carry
child: Mullein
Emotional ups and downs:
Chamomile
Energy protection: Yarrow
Miscarriage: Bleeding
Heart; *soothing of grief:*
Borage
Nausea and stomach upset:
Chamomile
Transition in each stage
of pregnancy: Walnut

Trauma or accident:
Five Flower Formula
Rescue Remedy
Unconscious destructive
intent toward child:
Evening Primrose
Weighed down:
Wild Potato Bush

CHILDBIRTH
Calm during:
Bougainvillea,
Five Flower Formula
Energy flow through sexual
organs: Macrozamia
Fear of child not being
healthy: Crowea
Joy and happiness: Valerian
Knowing what is needed
for yourself: Self-heal
Moving on to next stage
in labor: Sticky Geranium

Opening energy of spine:
Amazon Waterlily, Lilac
Pain relief: Wild Flower
Relief elixir, Pain Cream
Pressure buildup: Impatiens
Relaxing into the pain:
Sea Anemone
Releasing child: Walnut

BABY
Colic: Chamomile
Exhausted from birth: Olive
First steps:
Wild Potato Bush
Overstimulated:
Fairy Duster
Recovery from birth, for
mother or child: Fireweed
Sleep: Chamomile,
Fairy Duster, Sea
Anemone, Yarrow
Unsettled: Chamomile

ABOVE *Flower essences can*
give support as you move
through life's stages.

MOTHERING
Accepting new role: Walnut
Bonding, for mother and
child: Evening Primrose
Manipulating child for self:
Chicory
Overresponsibility: Zinnia
Recovery from difficult
or tiring birth: Fireweed,
Olive, Star of Bethlehem
Single mother issues,
time issues, finding
inner resources:
Single Mothers' Formula

FATHERING

Adjusting to change:
Walnut
Building family relationships:
Bush Gardenia
Doubting own capacities:
Larch
*Enjoying children for
who they are:*
Dampiera
*Negative self-image as
father:* Sunflower

**INFANTS AND
TODDLERS**

*Calming emotional
tension:* Chamomile

Psychic, sensitive children:
Yarrow
*Self-confidence in creative
expression:* Larch
Spontaneity: Larch
Starting new school:
Walnut

ADOLESCENCE

Confusion about goals:
Wild Oat
*Creative forces or sexual
forces in boys:* Larch; *in
girls:* She Oak
Crushes: Bleeding Heart
Delayed adolescence:
Sticky Geranium, Walnut

Relaxation: Zinnia.
*Romance, opening heart
and mind up to:* Bush
Gardenia; *recovery from;*
Menzies Banksia
Severe entanglements:
Black Kangaroo Paw
Vocation, finding: Wild Oat
*Work, tendency to
overwork:* Dandelion, Oak

MIDLIFE CRISIS

Awakening self to meaning:
Ash, Self-heal,
Detached view of life: Ash
Dissatisfaction with self:
Wild Oat

Identity crises:
Sunflower
Negative view of:
Self-heal
*Toxicity due to end
of menstrual flow:*
Crab Apple
*Rediscovery of delight
in living:* Valerian

OLD AGE

*Facing old injuries with
a willingness to heal:*
Fireweed
*Maintaining an
enthusiasm for life:* Wild
Rose

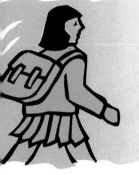

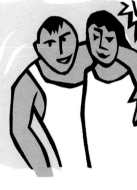

*Emotional neediness,
clinginess:* Chicory
Excessive attention-seeking:
Chicory
Fear of dark: St. John's Wort
Hyperactivity: Chamomile,
Fairy Duster
Jealousy: Chamomile, Holly
*Out of control, emotionally
or physically:*
Five Flower Formula
Overstimulation:
Fairy Duster
Teething: Chamomile,
Walnut
Temper tantrums: Chicory

SCHOOL AGE

Dreaming in class:
Clematis, Madia,
Fear of ridicule: Larch
Healthy sense of self:
Sunflower

Overall confidence: Larch
*Peer pressure,
withstanding:* Walnut
Rapid mood swings:
Chamomile
Self-confidence: Self-heal
Self-disgust (about spots):
Crab Apple
Study, focus: Madia;
*integrating new
information:* Fairy Duster

ADULTHOOD

Adapting to changes:
Walnut
Integration of self-hood:
Sunflower
Lack of maturation: Lilac
Perseverance toward goals:
Larch, Thyme
Potential, release into:
Sticky Geranium; *poor
expectation:* Larch

*Need to deepen knowledge
of self:* Himalayan Slipper
Orchid
*Need to make breaks with
past:* Bleeding Heart,
Walnut
Need to release past shock:
Star of Bethlehem
Overachievement, stress of:
Dandelion
*Reconsidering materialistic
values:* Honesty
*Unexplained feelings of
grief over what has not
been achieved:* Borage

MENOPAUSE

Celebration of: Zinnia
*Grief at cessation of
periods, especially if
childless:* Borage
*Grief concerning lack of
partner:* Bougainvillea

*Letting go of past
relationships:* Bleeding Heart
*Reverting to childish
behavior:* Chicory
Ripening to wisdom:
Amazon Waterlily
*Unnecessary fears about
health:* Apple

DEATH

*Going with the powerful
process:* Amazon Waterlily
*Grief over death of loved
ones:* Borage
Letting go: Dampiera
Seeing the light within:
St. John's Wort
Spiritual emergency:
St. John's Wort
Transformation:
Amazon Waterlily
When others cling on:
Walnut

Relationships Index

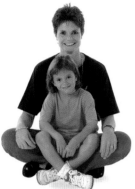

THIS IS AN INDEX *of themes that crop up in close relationships, since it is with others that we discover the wellsprings and the difficulties of our feelings. You may find when reading this list that you want your partner to take a particular essence. However, remember that you can't change anyone else, only yourself. Use the 49 essences in this book to help enrich and harmonize your intimate relationships. Give them time to work.*

ABOVE *Essences help bring harmony to close relationships*

A

Abandonment, fears of:
Evening Primrose, Rock Rose

Abuse, history of:
Cherry Plum,
Evening Primrose,
Fireweed, Macrozamia,
Star of Bethlehem, Walnut

Aggression:
Black Kangaroo Paw, Holly

Anxiety, about wanting everything to be perfect:
Dampiera; **about attaching:**
Evening Primrose; **about making new relationships:**
Menzies Banksia; **about sexuality:** Macrozamia

Attachment, over: Chicory;
not capable of making:
Evening Primrose

Argumentativeness, calming: Chamomile, Impatiens

Awareness, lack of:
Bush Gardenia, Clematis

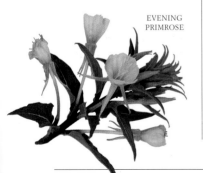

EVENING PRIMROSE

B

Bitterness:
Black Kangaroo Paw

Blocked emotions:
Dandelion, Sea Anemone,
blocked self-expression:
Larch, Star of Bethlehem

Broken-heartedness:
Bleeding Heart,
Borage, Chamomile,
Star of Bethlehem

C

Communication with partner: Bush Gardenia;
able to express self: Larch;
with honesty: Mullein

Compassion, for opposite sex: Macrozamia

Conflict: Bush Gardenia;
catalyst for peace: Holly;
for resolution through humor: Valerian

Confusion: Mullein

Control: Chicory

Criticism: Impatiens

D

Death, grief:
Menzies Banksia,
Star of Bethlehem

Deception: Mullein

Divorce, pain over:
Bleeding Heart;
surviving cheerfully:
Borage

Defenses to intimacy, hysterical: Fairy Duster;
overdeveloped:
Dampiera,
Evening Primrose,
Menzies Banksia

Dependency, and being demanding: Chicory

Depression about, abandonment:
Evening Primrose;
future of relationship:
Borage

Developmental arrest prevents growth of relationship: Lilac

Disillusionment:
Bush Gardenia

Domination:
Black Kangaroo Paw

Drained by others, absorbing physical and emotional imbalances:
Five Flower Formula,
Walnut

Drifting apart:
Bush Gardenia, Clematis,
Wild Rose

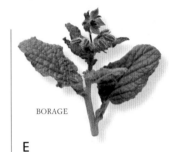

BORAGE

E

Emotional awareness, of self and others: Bougainvillea

Emotional pain:
Bleeding Heart;
upset: Chamomile;
turmoil: Five Flower Formula;
emotional suppression or distancing: Evening Primrose

Empathy, taking time to develop: Bush Gardenia;
opening up to: Bougainvillea

F

False self, interferes with forming true bond:
Mullein, Valerian

Fear of starting a new relationship: Menzies Banksia

Feelings, fear of expressing:
Larch; **overwhelming:**
Fairy Duster

Forgiveness:
Black Kangaroo Paw,
Fireweed

Freedom, need to allow others: Bleeding Heart

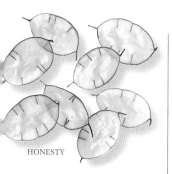

HONESTY

G

Greed: Honesty

H

Hate:
Black Kangaroo Paw, Holly

Holding on: Bleeding Heart

I

Idealization: Sunflower

Immaturity: Chicory, Lilac

Impatience:
Chamomile, Impatiens

Incest recovery:
Evening Primrose,
Fireweed, Macrozamia;
for male: Sunflower;
for female: Evening Primrose,
Five Flower Formula

Insecurity: Chicory

Insensitivity: Bush Gardenia

Insincerity: Honesty, Mullein

Intolerance:
Black Kangaroo Paw,
Bush Gardenia, Crab Apple,
Holly

Irritability:
Black Kangaroo Paw,
Chamomile

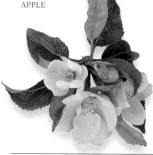

APPLE

J

Joy: Bougainvillea, Valerian,
Zinnia

L

Lack of self-esteem:
Sunflower, Larch

Letting go of loss:
Bleeding Heart, Dampiera,
Star of Bethlehem, Walnut

Love, all aspects:
Bush Gardenia;
opening up to: Holly

M

Manipulation:
Black Kangaroo Paw,
Chicory

Marriage, for all aspects of:
Bush Gardenia;
enjoyment of: Valerian

N

Neediness: Chicory, Valerian

O

**Obsessive need to get
attention:** Chicory

Openness: Sea Anemone

Overattachment:
Bleeding Heart;
controlling: Chicory

P

Passion, to renew:
Bush Gardenia

Peaceful relations: Holly

R

Receptivity, to love:
Bush Gardenia, Holly;
to the feelings of others:
Holly

Rejection:
Evening Primrose

**Renewal of intimacy, of
interest:** Dampiera

Resentment:
Black Kangaroo Paw,
Chicory

**Respect for another's
feelings:**
Black Kangaroo Paw, Holly;
for another's space: Chicory

Revenge:
Black Kangaroo Paw

S

Sadism:
Black Kangaroo Paw

Self-blame: Larch;
self-centered: Bush Gardenia;
self-depreciation:
Bougainvillea

Sensitivity, to increase:
Bush Gardenia

**Sexuality, over, or under
sexual:** Macrozamia;
**needs everything to be
perfect:** Dampiera;
to renew sensuality:
Bush Gardenia;
sexual repression:
Evening Primrose;
dryness during: She Oak

Solace:
Star of Bethlehem,
Valerian

Spontaneity: Valerian,
Zinnia

Stale relationships:
Bush Gardenia

Strengthen relationship:
Black Kangaroo Paw,
Bleeding Heart,
Evening Primrose

T

Taking for granted:
Bush Gardenia

Transformation:
Black Kangaroo Paw,
Sticky Geranium, Walnut

Trust, in partner:
Evening Primrose;
in self: Mullein

U

Unawareness:
Bush Gardenia, Clematis

Unconditional love: Chicory

Understanding:
Bougainvillea, Holly,
Impatiens

Unfulfilled: Bleeding Heart,
Dampiera, Macrozamia,
Wild Oat

Unproductive behavior:
Black Kangaroo Paw

**Unrecognized emotional
neediness:** Bleeding Heart

Unresolved conflict: Holly

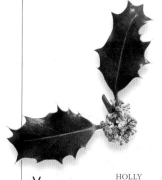

HOLLY

V

**Vulnerable to invasion by
thoughts, feelings of others:**
Walnut, Yarrow

W

Will-to-good: Apple

Willfulness:
Ash, Black Kangaroo Paw,
Chicory

**Worry, prevents relaxation
with partner:** Crowea;
about money issues: Honesty

**Wounds, uncovering
to heal:** Fireweed,
Star of Bethlehem

Self-help Index

THIS INDEX *is a list of broad categories that don't fit under the headings of life cycle, relationships, or emergencies. If you don't find what you need here, turn to these other sections. Once you have found the appropriate key word, look at the pages for the individual flowers suggested. You will probably know immediately whether that flower is right for you.*

ABOVE *Sunflower essence is useful for competitiveness.*

A

Achievement: Oak, Thyme

Abundance renewed:
Fireweed;
of spirit: Bougainvillea

Acceptance of circumstances: Dampiera

Adaptability: Ash,
Sea Anemone, Walnut

Aggression, replaced by positive masculine identity:
Sunflower

Aims: Madia, Self-heal,
Silver Princess, Wild Oat

Anger, overcoming:
Black Kangaroo Paw;
releasing: Lilac

Anxiety, general: Crowea;
about little things: Dampiera;
intense: Fairy Duster;
emotional: Chamomile;
about darkness:
St. John's Wort;
chronic: Garlic

Apathy about healing:
Fireweed, Wild Rose

Arrogance: Sunflower

Awareness of self:
Bougainvillea,
Himalayan Slipper Orchid

Avoidance: Wild Rose

B

Balance, for fulfilling needs:
Fairy Duster;
expression of masculine in men or women: Sunflower;
energetic: Crowea

Bitterness:
Black Kangaroo Paw,
Chicory, Holly

Bravery: Borage, Fireweed,
Garlic, Rock Rose

C

Calming, emotions:
Chamomile;
to get perspective: Ash;
to understand self and others: Bougainvillea;
to release negativity:
Black Kangaroo Paw;
to let go of hangups:
Dampiera;
during all kinds of stress:
Fairy Duster;
during health crises:
Apple

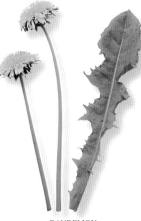

DANDELION

Centering: Madia,
Self-heal, Thyme

Character development:
Himalayan Slipper Orchid,
Lilac

Cheerfulness: Borage,
Zinnia

Childhood, clearing trauma:
Fireweed, Lilac, Self-heal,
Star of Bethlehem, Valerian

Choices, how to get well:
Self-heal;
life choices: Ash

Clarity, of purpose: Wild Oat;
of healing direction: Self-heal;
of values: Ash, Mullein;
of energy: Fairy Duster;
of focus: Madia

Compassion:
Black Kangaroo Paw, Holly

Competitiveness:
Sea Anemone, Sunflower

Completion: Clematis,
Madia, Walnut

Confidence, about future:
Borage;
self-confidence: Larch

Conflict, with others:
Bush Gardenia;
and confusion: Mullein;
about healing direction:
Self-heal

Conscience, to develop:
Mullein

Containment:
St. John's Wort, Yarrow

Contentment: Impatiens,
Wild Oat

Controlling attitudes:
Black Kangaroo Paw,
Dandelion

Courage: Borage, Rock Rose

Creativity, actualizing:
Clematis;

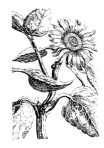

THYME

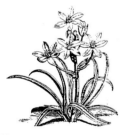
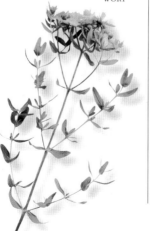
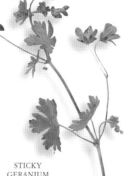
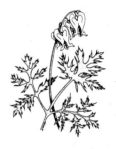

Inspiration, sense of wonder: Bougainvillea; **by spirit:** Amazon Waterlily

Integration, of emotions: Dandelion; **of personality:** Sunflower; **of subtle body:** Star of Bethlehem

Integrity: Mullein, Thyme

Intolerance: Crab Apple

Intuition: Self-heal; **about needs for life:** Ash

Irritability: Chamomile, Zinnia

Isolation: Evening Primrose, Zinnia

J

Joy of heart: Borage; **joyful enthusiasm:** Silver Princess; **joy of life:** Bougainvillea

Judgment of self: Bougainvillea

K

Kindness: Honesty

L

Learning processes: Clematis, Fairy Duster, Madia

Letting go, of troubled feelings: Chamomile; **of physical tension:** Dandelion; **of illness:** Self-heal; **of anything:** Dampiera

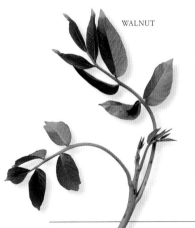

WALNUT

Life direction: Silver Princess, Walnut, Wild Oat

Light – strengthening one's inner light: Yarrow

Limitation – going beyond previous levels of self-definition: Sticky Geranium

Listening: Impatiens

Loneliness: Chicory, Dampiera, Valerian, Zinnia

Loss: Bleeding Heart, Star of Bethlehem, Walnut, Zinnia

Love, freely given to others: Chicory,

M

Masculine balance: Macrozamia, Sunflower

Materialism: Honesty

Meditation: Chamomile, Self-heal

Mental pain: Cherry Plum, Impatiens, Menzies Banksia

Moodiness: Chamomile

Motivation, to live life fully: Wild Rose; **to formulate goals:** Silver Princess; **to realize goals:** Clematis

N

Neediness: Chicory

Nervous breakdown: Fairy Duster

Night fears: Chamomile, St. John's Wort

Nourishment, for the heart: Borage; **for healing:** Self-heal; **for inner self:** Himalayan Slipper Orchid

Nurturing: Chicory, Olive, Self-heal

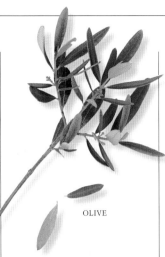

OLIVE

O

Obsession, with cleanliness: Crab Apple; **with fear:** Rock Rose; **with negativity:** Black Kangaroo Paw

Opening, the mind: Dampiera

Overwhelmed, by feelings: Chamomile; **by impressions and activities:** Fairy Duster; **by others:** Yarrow; **by emotional pain:** Menzies Banksia; **by terror:** Rock Rose

Overachieving: Oak, Sea Anemone

Overstimulation: Fairy Duster

Oversensitivity, to atmosphere: Yarrow; **to others:** Walnut

P

Past, recovery from past trauma: Fireweed, Star of Bethlehem, Walnut

Patience: Chamomile

Perfectionism: Bougainvillea

Perseverance: Borage, Dandelion, Oak

Perspective: Ash, Walnut

Positivity, when afraid: Borage; **toward life as a whole:** Wild Rose; **when in self-doubt:** Larch; **when ill:** Apple, Self-heal; **when overworked:** Valerian; **when losing direction:** Silver Princess; **when stuck:** Lilac, Sticky Geranium; **in deep grief:** Bougainvillea

Potential, releasing: Sticky Geranium; **harnessing in one direction:** Wild Oat; **releasing hidden:** Larch

Procrastination: Clematis, Sticky Geranium

Purification: Amazon Waterlily, Crab Apple

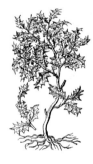

R

Rape, or abuse, recovery: Fireweed, Macrozamia, Star of Bethlehem

Rebelliousness: Silver Princess

Receptivity to enjoyment: Zinnia; **to higher frequencies:** Amazon Waterlily; **to creating sacred space:** Amazon Waterlily; **to environmental healing forces:** Fireweed; **to love:** Chicory, Holly; **to human bonding:** Evening Primrose

Regeneration: Fireweed

Rejection:
Evening Primrose

Rejuvenation: Fireweed,
Olive, Zinnia

Relaxation:
Chamomile, Dandelion,
Impatiens, Lilac, Oak,
Star of Bethlehem

Release, of painful feelings:
Chamomile;
of devastating past: Fireweed,
Star of Bethlehem;
into the future:
Sticky Geranium;
**from overinfluence
by others:** Walnut;
of tension: Dandelion;
from resistance, stagnation:
Lilac;
of fear: Rock Rose

Resilience:
Chamomile, Oak, Olive.

Resignation: Wild Rose

Restlessness: Wild Oat

S

Seeing: Sea Anemone

Shame, feeling contaminated:
Bougainvillea, Crab Apple;
**paralyzed by fear
of being shamed:** Larch;
shaming others: Larch

Shyness: Bush Gardenia,
Evening Primrose, Self-heal

Solitude, spiritual:
Amazon Waterlily

Soothing: Chamomile,
Star of Bethlehem

Spiritual, love:
Bougainvillea;
direction: Ash;
**taking care of spiritual
needs:** Honesty;
evolution: Crab Apple;
discipline:
Amazon Waterlily;

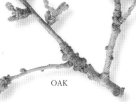

OAK

spiritual uplift:
Bougainvillea;
quest:
Himalyan Slipper Orchid

Strengthening, one's heart:
Borage;
one's inner light: Yarrow;
purpose: Silver Princess,
Thyme

Stress: Chamomile,
Dampiera, Dandelion,
Fairy Duster, Impatiens,
Sea Anemone, Yarrow

Stubbornness:
Fireweed, Oak, Self-heal

Sunny disposition:
Chamomile

Support, from others:
Bush Gardenia, Oak;
from healing forces in self:
Self-heal

**Surrender, upsetting
emotions:** Chamomile;
to higher forces:
Amazon Waterlily;
to relaxation: Dandelion;

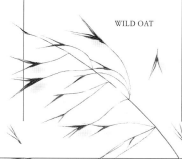

WILD OAT

to higher will: Rock Rose;
to past shocks:
Star of Bethlehem

Survival, after devastation:
Fireweed;
of deprivation:
Evening Primrose;
**after long drawn-out
struggle:** Oak, Olive

T

Tearfulness: Borage,
Chamomile, Chicory

Tension: Chamomile,
Dandelion, Impatiens

Tonic: Amazon Waterlily,
Olive

Transcendence:
Cherry Plum, Rock Rose,
Wild Potato Bush

Transformation: Fireweed

Transition: Walnut

Trauma, to resolve issues:
Fireweed;
to express without distress:
Chamomile;
courage to deal with:
Borage;
to resolve sexual traumas:
Macrozamia; **to deal with
shame connected with
sexual trauma:** Crab Apple;
to uncover and let go:
Star of Bethlehem

Trust in divine providence:
Honesty, Rock Rose,
St. John's Wort

Truthfulness: Mullein

U

Understanding:
Bush Gardenia,
Himalayan Slipper Orchid

Unhappiness:
Chicory, Valerian, Zinnia

Unfulfillment: Wild Oat

V

Values, being true to:
Mullein; **harmony with
spiritual nature:**
Amazon Waterlily, Ash

Vitality, of body: Oak,
Wild Potato Bush;
of spirit: Amazon Waterlily;
of will: Silver Princess, Thyme;
of energy body: Olive;
of health: Apple;
of focus: Madia;
of spine and nervous system:
Lilac;
**through balance of nervous
energy:** Fairy Duster;
through sense of freedom:
Zinnia

Vulnerability:
Garlic, St. John's Wort,
Thyme, Yarrow

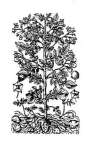

W

Warmth: Bush Gardenia,
Evening Primrose, Fireweed

Weighed down:
Oak, Wild Potato Bush

Will, to succeed: Larch;
to become purposeful:
Wild Oat;
toward achievement: Thyme;
to be well: Wild Rose

Wisdom, finding inner:
Himalayan Slipper Orchid,
Sticky Geranium

Worry: Borage, Chamomile,
Crowea, Dandelion

Y

Youthfulness: Olive, Zinnia

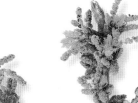

Using Flower Essences for Physical Ailments

MOST FLOWER *essence-makers would agree that flower essences do not directly heal physical ailments. Flower essence therapy treats you, not the problem. It is holistic medicine. An important principle of holistic medicine is that it honors your own healing ability. Flower essence therapy aids physical healing by supporting you to come to terms with and release the blocks to mental, emotional, and spiritual health that lie at the root of your inability to cope with your problem. It enhances your vitality to throw off disease by helping you to become more yourself, more in tune with your unique potential for good health, happiness, and fulfilment.*

The essences described here are only suggestions for you to explore. They are intended to help you explore the negative attitude or process that helped to cause the condition. A flower essence may have a strong physical impact at first and relieve pain, stress, and many other difficulties, but permanent relief comes through the flower essences' ability to reeducate us.

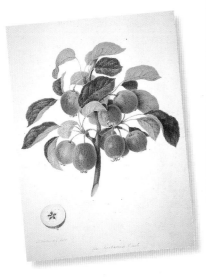

LEFT *Essences such as Crab Apple work on the mind as well as the body.*

EXAMPLE 1

The case history for Crab Apple (*see p. 87*) describes how the essence worked and how it cleared Hannah's skin rash but also how she had become fully aware of the shameful feelings she had been harboring. Through taking the essence, Hannah was able to make connections between her sense of shame about her rash and the painful experience she had had with her teacher. She let herself know that she didn't need to be physically perfect to be a good yoga teacher. Hannah was then able to overcome her need to hide her imperfections and talk to her flower essence practitioner. This was all part of her physical healing.

ABOVE *Walnut essence provides support in periods of change.*

EXAMPLE 2

The case history for Walnut essence (*see p. 73*) describes how it cured June's whooping cough. However, it is not a specific essence for that condition. Walnut suited the difficult transition with which the young girl was struggling. So it is important to take note not only of what strengths and weaknesses there are in your attitude, but also what particular support you might need at this time in your life.

A number of physical ailments are covered in the Emergency Essences Index (*see p. 127*). Where there are many suggestions, look them all up and find the one that best applies to your attitude. Check with a friend or therapist, if in doubt, or dowse. All the flower essences can be used as compresses, added to your bathwater, or applied directly to the body in creams.

A FLOWER ESSENCE HOME MEDICINE CHEST

Flower essences are absolutely safe to have in the home. The strength of the impact of a flower essence is due to repeated doses, therefore it is impossible to overdose. Taking a whole bottle at once would only work like one dose. The worst that could happen if, for instance, a child were to drink a whole dosage bottle over a day or two is that a healing or awareness crisis could occur but this is in no way dangerous (*see the case study for Walnut on p. 73*). In the same way, taking an essence too often, for too long, could only have as its worst effect a temporary worsening of moods. This would only serve to bring about greater awareness. Because

the flower essence has to be the right one to make any impact at all, you cannot make a dangerous diagnosis, only an ineffective one.

It is important to be aware that essences cannot take the place of consulting a physician or a qualified complementary practitioner. Flower essences can, however, help you become more aware of what is needed on an emotional level and thus ease physical pain and discomfort.

The most effective use of the essences is over a period of time to help you make any necessary changes in attitudes, and so gradually restore you to positive health and a vibrant love of life. Nonetheless the essences can

sometimes work very quickly and effectively, transforming what might be a miserable day into a worthwhile one in just one or two doses.

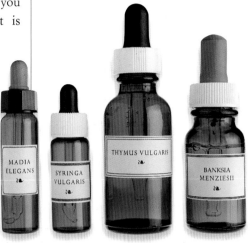

BELOW *Ensure that you have a supply of dosage bottles for your home medicine chest. They should be 1fl. oz (30ml) or larger.*

ESSENTIAL ITEMS FOR THE HOME

The following list is a suggestion for the essences and accessories that it would be useful to have in your home at all times.

Essential items for the home

❈ A supply of 1fl. oz. (30ml) dosage bottles

❈ Good natural water, such as uncarbonated spring water

❈ Base cream or oil, such as lanolin or grapeseed oil

❈ Vaporizer or spray

❈ Cotton material, lint, or flannel for compresses; hot water bottle for keeping compress warm

❈ Q-tips for direct application

❈ A stock bottle of an emergency essence appropriate to your part of the world

❈ Self-heal cream

❈ Stock bottles of the following essences:

APPLE • *for health*

BORAGE • *for cheerfulness*

CHAMOMILE • *for calm emotions*

CRAB APPLE • *for cleansing*

CROWEA • *for feeling balanced*

DANDELION • *for relaxing body and mind*

GARLIC • *for feeling strong*

LARCH • *for feeling confident*

LILAC • *for being flexible*

MACROZAMIA • *for balancing male and female, within and without*

MADIA • *for focusing on your task*

MENZIES BANKSIA • *to let go of pain in relationships*

OLIVE • *for recuperation*

SEA ANEMONE • *for swimming with the tide*

SELF-HEAL • *for feeling confident and clear about your health*

ST. JOHN'S WORT • *for feeling light inside, good peaceful sleep*

THYME • *to support your immune system*

WALNUT • *to support you through all major and minor changes*

YARROW • *to protect you from harmful influences*

Glossary

Caduceus. A primal energetic force that created the human body. It consists of two magnetic serpentine currents, one negative, the other positive, that, as they cross each other, form five neutral energy centers at certain points in the body.

Chakras. Areas of pulsatory energy created at the points where the magnetically positive and negative currents of the caduceus cross. These chakras whirl like catherine wheels pushing energy out from the center, but unlike catherine wheels they also draw it back in. Each chakra relates to a primal force of nature called an element.

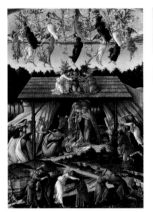

CHAKRA

Elements. The elements are the subtle equivalent of earth, water, fire, air, and ether (or space), in nature. You cannot see them operate but they behave in the body in much the same way that they do in nature.

The elements support or combat each other. For instance, in the same way that fire can evaporate water, laughter can dry out tears.

Holistic. Means whole and is derived from the Anglo-Saxon word *hele* meaning healing and wholeness. A holistic health care perspective focuses on fortifying the vitality of the emotional, mental, and spiritual aspects of a person to supplement or counterbalance the purely physiological approach of much modern medicine.

Luscher color test. This is used in many different settings – business and healing – to draw up personality profiles from a complex sequence of color selections. It is a very useful tool when we are puzzled by ourselves.

Meridian. This is a term from Chinese medicine given to the tiny pathways just below the surface of the skin that conduct energy or *chi* around the body. They are mirrored on each side of the body. Energy travels through the meridians in well-defined cycles that relate to the movement of the elements in the body and in nature.

Potency. Potency is the strength of a homeopathic remedy. The higher the number the greater the strength or potency, and the greater the dilution. Potentization is the process

SPIRIT

of diluting a small amount of a substance, which is then forcefully shaken or succussed in order to ensure the molecular "pattern" of the substance is spread throughout.

Shenmen point. Shen means Spirit; the Shen cycle is the creative movement of energy through the five elements. The Shenmen point on the ear relates to nerve control. With your finger in the dip under the upper part of the ear trace down the gristly ridge. The Shenmen point is about 2in. (5cm) down.

Spirit. Spirit can be expressed as the transcendent force – sometimes called God. It is the principle of consciousness that is in every animate being. The individual soul's yearning for wholeness and balance is one expression of the spirit. Flower essence therapy supports the spirit because the bloom is the expression of the plant's soul.

Subtle energy. Energy is the animating force within all phenomena. It is called subtle because generally it cannot be seen directly although it is the real substance behind the appearance of forms.

Succussion. The act of vigorously shaking a homeopathic remedy in order to give it potency.

Tincture. A tincture is made by macerating the relevant parts of the plant in alcohol (usually) for about two weeks, and then pressing and filtering the mixture.

Vibrational medicine. A group of healing modalities that in different ways work to integrate and balance the energetic body, mind, or spirit systems rather than using mechanical, chemical, or physical means. They include homeopathy, flower essence therapy, acupuncture, polarity therapy, cranial-sacral therapy, reiki healing, gem and crystal therapy.

Virtue. The "virtue" of a plant is the special quality that enables it to heal. It was considered so important to know these "virtues" that often the gods were said to have revealed them.

Useful Addresses

AUSTRALASIA

Bush Essences
8a Oaks Avenue,
Dee Why, NSW Australia.
Tel 61 2 9972 1033,
Fax 61 2 99721102.
(Training courses, suppliers)

Living Essences
Australian Flower Essence
Academy, PO Box 355,
Scarborough 6019, Perth,
Western Australia.
(Training courses, suppliers)

Martin & Pleasance
137 Swan Street,
Richmond Victoria 3121,
Australia.
Tel 61 2 6139 427 7422
(Suppliers)

**New Perception
Flower Essences**
Mary and Dolf Garbely,
PO Box 60-127 Titirangi,
Auckland 1230, New Zealand.
Tel/fax 64 9 817 775.
(Training courses, suppliers)

U.S.A. & CANADA

**Alaskan Flower Essence
Project**
PO Box 1369,
Homer, Alaska 99603.
(Suppliers)

Desert Alchemy
PO Box 44189,
Tucson AZ 85733.
Tel 1 520 325 1545,
fax 1 520 325 8405.
(Training courses, suppliers)

Flower Essence Society,
PO Box 459,
Nevada City, CA 95959.
Tel 800 736 9222 or
530 265 9163,
fax 530 265 0584.
(Research, training courses)

Flower Essence Services,
PO Box 1769,
Nevada City, CA 95959.
Tel 800 548 0075 or
530 2650258,
fax 530 265 6467.
(Suppliers)

**Hawaiian Tropical Flower
Essences**
Aloha Flower Essences Inc.
PO Box 2319, Kealakekua,
Hawaii 96750.
Fax 808 328 2529.
(Suppliers)

Masters Flower Essences
141618 Tyler-Foote Road,
Nevada City, CA 95959.
Tel 916 478 7655,
Toll free ordering:
800 347 3639.
(Training courses, suppliers)

Nelson Bach U.S.A. Ltd.
Wilmington Technology Park,
100 Research Drive, Wilmington,
Massachusetts 01887 4406.
Tel 978 988 3833.
fax 978 988 0233.
(Suppliers)

Pacific Essences
Box 8317, Victoria,
BC V8W 3R9, Canada.
Tel 250 384 5560,
Fax 250 595 7700.
(Training courses, suppliers)

**Perelandra, Center for
Nature Research**
PO Box 3603,
Warrenton, VA 20188.
Tel 800 960 8806 or
540 937 2153,
fax 540 937 3360.
(Training courses, suppliers)

Petite Fleur Essences,
Herbal Essence, Inc,
Box 330411, Fort Worth,
Texas 76163. (Suppliers)

EUROPE

Aquarius Flower Remedies
Threpwood Hill Cottage,
Birtley Nr. Wark, Hexham,
NE48 3HI, England.
Tel 44 1434 230499.
(Training courses, suppliers)

Bailey Essences
7/8 Nelson Road, Ilkley,
West Yorkshire,
LS29 8HN, England.
Tel 44 1943 432012,
fax 44 1943 432011.
(Suppliers)

Deva, Elixirs Floraux Deva
La Laboratoire Deva,
BP3, 38880 Autrans, France.
Tel 33 76 95 35 87,
fax 33 76 95 37 02.
(Training courses, suppliers)

Bach Flower Remedies
Dr. Edward Bach Centre,
Mount Vernon, Sotwell,
Wallingford, Oxon
OX10 0PZ, England.
Tel 44 1491 834678,
fax 44 1491 825022.
(Training courses, suppliers)

Findhorn Flower Essences
Mercury, Findhorn Bay, Forres,
Moray, Scotland IV36 OTY.
Tel 44 1309 690129,
fax 44 139 690933.
(Suppliers)

Harebell Remedies
PO Box 7536, Dumfries
DG2 7DZ, SW Scotland.
Tel 44 1387 261962.
(Counseling, suppliers)

Healing Herbs Ltd
The Flower Remedy
Programme, PO Box 65,
Hereford HR2 OUW,
England.
Tel 44 1873 890218.
(Suppliers)

**Andreas Korte/Korte Phi
Essences**
Haupstrasse 9, D-78267
Aach, Germany.
Tel 49 77 74 70 04,
fax 49 7774 70 09.
Distributed by PHI
Interservices SA, 19a rue de
la Croix d'Or, Switzerland.
Tel 41 22 331 03 22,
fax 41 22 331 04 20.
(Training courses, suppliers)

**Dutch Flower Essences/
Bloesem Remedies
Nederland**
St Jansstraat 3, 5964 AA
Horst, Netherlands.
Tel 31 077 3987826,
fax 31 077 3987826.
(Training courses, suppliers)

Green Man Tree Essences
Simon and Sue Lilly,
2 Kerswell Cottages,
Exminster, Exeter, Devon
EX6 8AY, England.
Tel 44 1392 832005
(Suppliers)

**International Flower
Essence Repertoire**
The Working Tree,
Milland, Liphook, Hants,
GU30 7JS. England.
Tel 44 1428 741 572,
fax 44 1428 741 679.
(Training courses, suppliers)

Carol Rudd
Dancing Man, Burgh Hall,
Aylsham, Norfolk,
NR11 6TD, England.
Tel/fax 44 1263 732523.
(Training courses, counseling)

**Unitive Flower and Life
Essences,** Dr. Maria Thaw,
Cynlas, Rhos Isaf,Caenarfon,
Gwynedd, LL54 7NL, Wales.
Tel 44 1286 830555.
(Suppliers)

Bibliography

Amodeo, J., and Amodeo, K., *Being Intimate – A Guide to Successful Relationships,* Arkana, 1993.

Bailey, A., *Dowsing for Health,* Quantum, 1990.

Bailey, A., *The Bailey Flower Essences Handbook,* Quantum, 1992.

Barnao, Dr. V., and Barnao, Dr. K., *Walkabout Healing Handbook, Healing with the Living Essences of Australian Flowers,* Australasian Flower Essence Academy, 1990.

Barnard, J. (ed), *The Collected Writings of Dr. Bach,* Bach Educational Programme, 1987.

Barnard, J., *Patterns of Life Force,* Bach Educational Programme, 1987.

Barnard, J., and Barnard, M. *The Healing Herbs of Edward Bach: A Practical Guide to Making the Remedies,* Bach Educational Programme, 1988.

OENOTHERA HOOKERI

Blamey, M. and Grey-Wilson, C., *The Illustrated Flora of Britain and Northern Europe,* Hodder & Stoughton, 1989.

Bowers, J. E., *Shrubs and Trees of the Southwest Deserts,* Southwest Parks and Monuments Association, 1993.

Bradshaw, J., *Healing the Shame that Binds You,* Piatkus, 1998.

Bradshaw, J., *Home Coming, Reclaiming and Championing Your Inner Child,* Piatkus, 1990.

Bremness, L., *The Complete Book of Herbs,* Dorling Kindersley, 1996.

Bricknell, C., A–Z *Encyclopedia of Garden Plants,* Dorling Kindersley, 1996.

Bruce-Mitford, M., *The Illustrated Book of Signs and Symbols,* Dorling Kindersley, 1996.

Chase, P. L., and Pawlik, J., *Trees for Healing,* Newcastle Publishing Co. Inc., 1991.

Devi, L., *The Essential Flower Essence Handbook,* Masters Flower Essences, 1996.

Edlin, H. L., and Nimmo, M., *The World of Trees,* Orbis Publishing, 1974.

Gibbons, B., and Brough, P., *The Hamlyn Photographic Guide to the Wild Flowers of Britain and Northern Europe,* Hamlyn, 1992.

Gimbel, T., *The Book of Color Healing,* Gaia Books, 1994.

Grieve, M., *A Modern Herbal,* Jonathan Cape, 1979.

Griffin, J., *Returning to the Source* and *Romancing the Rose,* Herbal Essence Inc., 1984.

Griffin, J., *Mother Nature's Herbal,* Llewellyn Publications, 1997.

Harris, T. Y., *Wild Flowers of Australia,* Angus and Robertson, 1948.

Harvey, C. G., and Cochrane, A., *The Encyclopedia of Flower Remedies,* Thorsons, 1995.

Heywood, V. H. *Flowering Plants of the World,* B. T. Batsford Ltd., 1993.

Hoffmann, David, *The Complete Illustrated Holistic Herbal,* Element Books, 1996.

Hopman, E. E., *Tree Medicine Tree Magic,* Phoenix Publishing Inc., 1992.

Johnson, H., *The International Book of Trees,* Simon and Schuster, 1977.

Johnson, S., *The Essence of Healing, A Guide to the Alaskan Flower, Gem, and Environmental Essences,* Alaskan Flower Essence Project, 1996.

Kaminski, P. and Katz, R., *Affirmations, the Messages of the Flowers in Transformative Words for the Soul,* F.E.S., 1994.

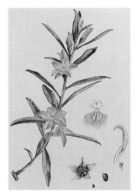

CROWEA SALIGNA

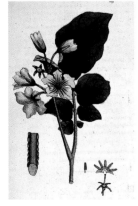

SOLANUM QUADRILOCULATUM

Kaminski, P. and Katz, R.,
*Flower Essence Repertory,
A Comprehensive Guide to
North American* and *English
Flower Essences for Emotional
and Spiritual Well-Being,*
F.E.S., U.S.A., 1994.

Kaplan-Williams, S.,
The Elements of Dreamwork,
Element Books, 1990.

Kemp, C. A., *Cactus and
Company, Patterns and
Qualities of Desert Alchemy
Flower Essences,*
Desert Alchemy, 1993.

Korte, A.,
*Orchids, Gemstones and
Their Healing Energies,*
Bauer Verlag, 1997, and
Findhorn Press.

Kramer, D.,
*New Bach Flower Therapies,
Healing the emotional and
spiritual causes of illness,*
Healing Arts Press, 1995.

Kramer, K. and Wild, H.,
*New Bach Flower Body
Maps, Treatment by
Topical Application,*
Healing Arts Press, 1996.

Lavender, S. and Franklin, A.,
*Herb Craft: A Guide to the
Shamanic and Ritual
Use of Herbs,*
Capall Bann, 1996.

Lawless, Julia,
*The Complete Illustrated
Guide to Aromatherapy,*
Element Books, 1997.

Lawless, Julia, *The Illustrated
Encyclopedia of Essential Oils,*
Element Books, 1995.

LeShan, L., *Holistic Health,
How to Understand and Use
the Revolution in Medicine,*
Turnstone Press, 1997.

LeShan, L.,
*How to Meditate,
A Guide to Self Discovery,*
Turnstone Press, 1993.

Medeiros, P.,
*Hawaiian Tropical Flower
Essences,* Aloha Flower
Essences, Inc., 1995.

Myss, C., *Anatomy of the
Spirit, The Seven Stages
of Power and Healing,*
Harmony Books, 1997.

Neal, B., *Gardener's Latin*,
Robert Hale Ltd., 1992.

Ody, P., *The Herb Society's
Complete Medicinal Herbal,*
Dorling Kindersley, 1993.

Paterson, J. M.,
*Tree Wisdom: The Definitive
Guidebook to the Myth,
Folklore, and Healing
Power of Trees,*
Thorsons, 1996.

Petit, S.,
*Energy Medicine, Pacific
Flower and Sea Essences,*
Pacific Essences, 1993.

Pierrakos, Dr. J.,
Core Energetics,
Life Rhythm, 1987.

Scott, I. (trans. and ed.),
The Luscher Test, Pan, 1970.

Shealy, C. N. (ed.),
*The Complete Family Guide
to Alternative Medicine,*
Element Books, 1996.

Sills, F. *The Polarity Process,
Energy as a Healing Art*,
Element Books, 1988.

Simpson, D. P.,
Cassell's Latin Dictionary,
Cassell, 1982.

Stearn, W. T. *Botanical Latin*,
Fourth Edition,
David and Charles, 1996.

Stone, Dr. R.,
*Polarity Therapy,
Volumes One and Two,*
CRCS Publications, 1987.

Sullivan, K. (ed.),
*The Complete Family Guide
to Natural Home Remedies,*
Element Books, 1997.

Veith, I. (trans.),
*The Yellow Emperor's
Classic of Internal Medicine,*
University of California
Press, Berkeley, 1956.

Weeks, N.,
*The Medical Discoveries of
Edward Bach, Physician,*
The C.W. Daniel Co. Ltd.,
1973.

White, I.,
Bush Flower Essences,
Bantam Press, 1991.

Wood, M.,
*The Magical Staff:
The Vitalist Tradition in
Western Medicine*,
North Atlantic Books, 1992.

Wright, M. S.,
Flower Essences,
Perelandra Ltd, 1988.

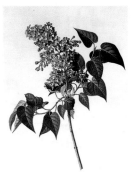

The deep purple Lilac.

SYRINGA VULGARIS

FRAXINUS EXCELSIOR

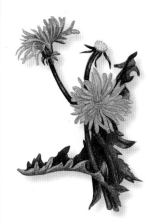

TARAXACUM OFFICINALE

Index